Don't Drink Your Milk!

The Frightening New Medical Facts About the World's Most Over-rated Nutrient.

by FRANK A OSKI, M.D.

TEACH Services, Inc.

Brushton, New York

Copyright © 1996 by TEACH Services, Inc.
Copyright © 1983 by Frank A. Oski

ISBN 0-945383-34-7
Library of Congress Catalog Number 77-8102

Published by

TEACH Services, Inc.
www.tsibooks.com

DEDICATED TO:

*Dr. Lewis A. Barness —
he was the first to teach me
that "cow milk is for calves."*

Table of Contents

Chapter 1

"Milk Is a Natural"

When my youngest daughter was in the second grade she came home one afternoon perplexed and teary-eyed. She had failed to get a perfect grade on her daily reading quiz. We reviewed the questions together. The quiz contained three questions designed to test reading comprehension and requiring simple "yes" and "no" answers.

Here were the test questions:

"Do you think a rabbit could make a mitten?"
"Can a fish hop like a rabbit?"
"Should all boys and girls have milk?"

To all three she had answered "no." The teacher had found her answer to the one about milk unacceptable and graded it as incorrect. Yet my daughter had been taught at home that people don't need cow milk and, in fact, that for many people it was actually harmful to their health. This information came as a surprise to her teacher who, I suspect, still believes I'm living on the lunatic fringe of society.

Being against cow milk is equated with being un-American. It is easy to understand this view, which is inspired mainly by the advertising practices and political pressure of the American dairy industry. For many of us, our earliest memories of childhood include our mother's plea, "Hurry up and finish your milk!" We have all been exposed to subtle endorsements of cow milk like that reading test given to my daughter and her fellow second graders, and we can all recite the industry's familiar slogans and jingles: "Milk is a Natural," "Milk is the Perfect Food," "Everybody Needs Milk," and you've probably seen the bumper sticker, "Milk Drinkers Make Better Lovers."

This advertising has been remarkably successful. One dollar of every seven spent for food in the United States goes for the purchase of milk and milk products. Each person in this country consumes, on the average, 375 pounds of dairy products each year. These items make up the second largest food expense, ranking behind only the combined expenses for meat, fish, poultry, and eggs. Eighteen million cows in the United States tell us by their rotund reality, "The dairy industry is big business." This agglomerate carries solid political punch: from it, one of every seven members of Congress receives support for re-election. Milk producers' cooperatives exert legislative pressures to artificially maintain high prices for milk; they benefit from many state and federal laws, and tax their farmer-members as much as five cents per hundred pounds of milk produced to continue all forms of milk promotion. Thomas V. Angott, chairman of the National Dairy Council, took pride in telling members, "Milk sales" stayed up during the recent recession," even in areas of high unemployment such as

Detroit, thanks to the effective milk promotion efforts of the industry.

But at last a growing number of physicians, private citizens and even the Federal Trade Commission are beginning to re-examine these long standing and deeply ingrained beliefs in the virtue of cow milk. And even Richard Nixon and John Connally came to realize that cow milk may not be good for you.

The fact is: the drinking of cow milk has been linked to iron-deficiency anemia in infants and children; it has been named as the cause of cramps and diarrhea in much of the world's population, and the cause of multiple forms of allergy as well; and the possibility has been raised that it may play a central role in the origins of atherosclerosis and heart attacks.

Among physicians, so much concern has been voiced about the potential hazards of cow milk that the Committee on Nutrition of the prestigious American Academy of Pediatrics, the institutional voice of practicing pediatricians, released a report entitled, "Should Milk Drinking by Children Be Discouraged?" Although the Academy's answer to this question has (as of this writing) been a qualified "maybe," the fact that the question was raised at all is testimony to the growing concern about this product, which for so long was viewed as sacred as the proverbial goodness of mother and apple pie.

Most lay persons are not aware that the milk of mammalian species varies considerably in its composition. For example, the milk of goats, elephants, cows, camels, yaks, wolves, and walruses show marked differences, one from the other, in their content of fats, protein, sugar, and minerals. Each was designed to provide optimum nutrition to the young

3

of the respective species. Each is different from human milk.

In general, most animals are exclusively breast-fed until they have tripled their birth weight, which in human infants occurs around the age of one year. In no mammalian species, except for the human (and the domestic cat), is milk consumption continued after the weaning period. Calves thrive on cow milk. Cow milk is for calves.

In many other parts of the world, most particularly in East Asia, Africa, and South America, people regard cow milk as unfit for consumption by adult human beings. If we are to judge by general mammalian standards their tastes are not peculiar; Americans' and Europeans' tastes are. Despite our notions, it is not the Chinese and Africans who differ most markedly from the norms of nature.

Cow milk, like all milks, contains three basic ingredients—sugar, fat, and protein. These three substances are suspended in water that also contains a variety of minerals and vitamins. Each of the three basic ingredients of cow milk has now come under scrutiny as a cause of problems in human nutrition.

The Federal Trade Commission in April, 1974, issued a "proposed complaint" against the California Milk Producers Advisory Board and their advertising agency. In this complaint they cited the slogan "Everybody Needs Milk" as representing false, misleading, and deceptive advertising. The Federal Trade Commission judged that enthusiastic testimonials by celebrities such as Olympic swimmer Mark Spitz, baseball pitcher Vida Blue, dancer Ray Bolger, columnist Abigail Van Buren, and singer Florence Henderson conveyed an inaccurate picture of the value of milk as a food. Quickly the dairymen changed their approach and came up with a new slogan: "Milk

Has Something for Everybody." This is certainly technically correct. The question you must ask yourself before you drink that next glass of milk, however, is: do you really want that "something?"

Lactose Intolerance

Chapter 2

"Fifty Cents for a Quart of Intestinal Gas!

Mrs Edwards was forty years old when her only son was sent to Vietnam. Mrs. Edwards had been widowed when her husband, a police officer, was killed in a gun battle with a gang of thieves. She worried that her son, age nineteen, might also die from gunfire. As the intensity of the war in Vietnam increased and her son's letters became more infrequent she began to experience vague and recurrent pains in her upper abdomen. After a while the pains awakened her at night. Sharpening, the pains were associated with tenderness to the touch in an area midway between her breastbone and her navel.

Finally this "heartburn" forced her to see her family physician. The doctor, after listening to Mrs. Edwards story, suspected that she had developed an ulcer and sent her to a local hospital for some X-rays of her stomach and upper gastrointestinal tract. The studies revealed that Mrs. Edwards did in fact have a duodenal ulcer. The doctor prescribed some medication and also instructed Mrs. Edwards to drink large quantities of milk. She was to drink a glass between breakfast and lunch, a glass with lunch, a glass in the mid-afternoon, another with dinner, and a final glass at bedtime. She followed this schedule carefully, and within a matter of several weeks her stomach pains vanished. But now Mrs. Edwards was experiencing another form of discomfort. Constantly bloated, she had intermittent cramps in her lower abdomen, passed watery stools, and was continually embarrassed by the expulsion of large volumes of gas by rectum.

Mrs. Edwards returned to her doctor. He repeated the X-ray studies of her stomach and upper gastrointestinal tract. Her ulcer had been cured. The doctor told Mrs. Edwards that her present complaints were a sign of an "irritable colon" brought on by continued concern about her son and that if they persisted she would have to see a psychiatrist. He urged her to continue on her medication and her diet to prevent a recurrence of her ulcer.

By chance, Mrs. Edwards discussed her problem with a woman friend who had herself experienced the same complaints of lower abdominal cramps, bloating, and gas. Her friend's doctor had explained that she had "lactose intolerance" and that the symptoms were caused by the drinking of milk. When Mrs. Edwards heard this she decided that rather than go to a psychiatrist, she would stop drinking milk. It worked. Overnight her symptoms disappeared.

Mrs. Edwards' story is not unusual: milk consumption does produce gastrointestinal complaints. The majority of people in this world over four years old are, in fact, "lactose intolerant!"

What is lactose intolerance and what is its relationship to cow milk?

Lactose is the sugar in milk. It is the only sugar, also termed carbohydrate, present in milk. Lactose is a "disaccharide," meaning that it is made up of two simple sugars. Glucose and galactose are the two monosaccharides that, linked together, form the disaccharide lactose. This sugar is formed only by the cells of the lactating mammary gland; thus no other food except mammalian milk contains lactose. The only mammals that do not have lactose—or any other carbohydrate in their milk—are seals, sea lions, and walruses. Human milk contains about 75 grams of lactose per quart while cow milk contains close to 45 grams per quart.

When consumed in milk, lactose, the disaccharide, must be broken down into its two monosaccharides before it can be absorbed from the intestinal tract into the bloodstream. Lactase is the enzyme that breaks down the lactose in milk and milk products. Lactase is present in the intestinal cells of the upper part of the gastrointestinal tract and its highest concentration is in that portion of the small bowel called the jejunum.

Lactase activity first appears in the intestinal tract of infants during the last third of pregnancy and is at its height shortly after birth. If the amount of lactose in the diet exceeds the capacity of the lactase in the intestine to break it down, then the lactose is undigested and proceeds to the large intestine. When the undigested lactose reaches the colon, or large intestine, two things happen. First the lactose is acted upon by the bacteria that normally inhabit the colon. They ferment the lactose and convert it to a gas, car-

to counter act the acidity

bon dioxide, and to an acid, lactic acid. The lactose molecules also cause water to be drawn into the intestinal tract by a process of osmosis. As a result, more gas and water are present in the colon. This combination produces a sense of bloating and also results in belching, the passage of gas from the rectum, cramps, and may induce a watery diarrhea.

Prior to 1965 it was assumed that absence of lactase in the intestinal tract was an unusual disorder seen in some infants as a result of an hereditary abnormality; either that or it occurred in association with other diseases of the intestinal tract. It was in that year that investigators at the Johns Hopkins School of Medicine first observed that 15 percent of all whites and 70 percent of all blacks tested were unable to digest lactose. Surveys of the world populations were begun and we now know that far more people are unable to digest lactose than are able to digest it.

Sometime between the age of one and a half and four years most individuals gradually lose the lactase activity in their small intestine. This appears to be a normal process that accompanies maturation. It occurs in most mammals shortly after they are weaned. Humans behave just like other animals in this regard.

To give you some appreciation of how common lactase deficiency is, here are some statistics:

Prevalence of
Lactase Deficiency
Population Group in Healthy Adults

Bantus	90 percent
Thais	90 percent
Filipinos	90 percent
Greek Cypriots	85 percent
Japanese	85 percent
Taiwanese	85 percent
Greenland Eskimos	80 percent
Arabs	78 percent
Ashkenazic Jews	78 percent
(throughout the world)	
Peruvians	70 percent
American blacks	70 percent
Israeli Jews	58 percent
Indians	50 percent
Finns	18 percent
American whites	8 percent
Swiss	7 percent
Danes	2 percent

[handwritten note: milk ? to get vitamin D]

Since the majority of the people on earth are either black or yellow it is easy to see that that same majority are lactase-deficient. It might be guessed that if cow milk had not been white it would never have become popular in the first place.

Dr. Norman Kretchmer, Director of the Institute of Child Health and Human Development of the National Institutes of Health, several years ago analyzed the distribution of lactase deficiency in Nigeria. He studied four of the major tribal groups of that country—the Yoruba, Ibo, Hausa, and Fulani. The Yoruba and Ibo live in an area of the country where there is no cattle raising and where almost no milk is consumed after weaning. In these groups 99 percent of the population was lactase deficient between one and a half and three years of age. The Hausa and Fulani live in the north of Nigeria, where cattle raising and ingestion of milk and milk products is traditional. Among the nomadic dairy herders of the Fulani tribe, who live chiefly on milk and milk products, the incidence of lactase deficiency was only 20 percent.

Dr. Kretchmer concluded from these observations that the ability to absorb lactose was *genetically* determined and that a process of natural selection was responsible for the fact that tribes who must live from milk in order to survive developed a high incidence of mutant individuals who retained the presence of the enzyme lactase. It is natural to lose the lactase activity in the gastrointestinal tract. It is a biological accompaniment of growing up. Most people do it. All animals do it. It reflects the fact that nature never intended lactose-containing foods, such as milk, to be consumed after the normal weaning period. If loss of the enzyme lactase is the usual pattern of development, then those individuals who retain the capacity to digest this sugar after infancy might, in American slang, be called "milk freaks."

Prior to the recognition of lactase deficiency, the problems created by the shipment of powdered milk to the developing countries of the world were a source of puzzlement and frustration to U.S. government officials. Stories are now legend about what happened after initial shipments of powdered milk arrived in some South American countries. The natives carefully followed instructions concerning the reconstitution of the powdered milk with water. However, after the product became palatable and was drunk, widespread outbreaks of cramps and diarrhea were experienced in the villages.

Reaction was strong and widespread: "Another ingenious imperialist plot." When subsequent shipments of powdered milk were received the natives mixed them with far less water and then used it to whitewash their huts. Some American scientists believe that the U.S. dairy industry has been attempting to "whitewash" the entire lactase-deficiency problem ever since.

Unfortunately cow milk is still a staple of the government-sponsored school lunch programs. These programs are primarily supposed to benefit children in inner-city schools and are designed to provide students with at least one good meal per day. Most of these children in the major cities are black. A group of Johns Hopkins investigators observed the milk-drinking habits of 300 black and 200 white children in the Baltimore schools. At lunch, each child was given a half-pint of milk. The majority of the blacks consumed less than half their milk, with most drinking less than one-fourth. In contrast, only 10 percent of the whites failed to drink at least half their milk. When the latter children were tested for their ability to digest lactose it was found that among all white children 18 percent were unable to digest lactose while 33 percent of the black milk drinkers had abnormal tests and 77 percent of the non-milk drinkers had abnormal tests. When the black children who were non-milk drinkers were given lactose as a test, 85 percent of them developed symptoms of cramping pain, gas, or diarrhea.

These investigators concluded that lactose intolerance was a major factor in milk rejection among black children. Although these children had learned that milk drinking would lead to unpleasant consequences for them, the U.S. government is still acting as if it is unaware of the problem. Milk not only continues to be a key staple in these government-subsidized lunch programs, but even worse, additional funds were allocated and spent in 1976 for food supplement programs. In these programs, stamps can only be used for a limited number of foods; one of these items is milk.

The fact that many individuals are lactose-intolerant helps to explain what was once believed to be a cultural myth concerning the healing properties of yogurt and cheese. When milk is made into yogurt by incubating it with a bacterial stock, much of the lactose is broken down into glucose and galactose. Similarly, when cheese ripens, much of the lactose is also converted to simple sugars. These substances can now be tolerated by individuals who would be otherwise intolerant of whole milk.

The old expression that cheese or yogurt was "binding" probably reflects the fact that when lactase-deficient individuals switched to these products they noticed that their stools became firmer. Yogurt is frequently administered to infants with diarrhea. During the course of diarrhea many infants will experience a transient lactase deficiency. When this occurs, the continual administration of milk only aggravates the gastrointestinal upset. Because this phenomenon is so common, American manufacturers of baby formulas have produced lactose-free milks to be used when feeding is resumed in infants afflicted with diarrhea.

The dairy industry has openly criticized the findings of the lactose tolerance tests. Spokesmen contend, "The amounts of lactose administered in the tests are unusually large and thus have no bearing on what might be expected to occur with more normal milk consumption. While it is true that lactose intolerance should not be equated with milk intolerance, tests have demonstrated that as many as 60 to 75 percent of individuals judged to be lactase-deficient by conventional testing, will experience gastrointestinal upsets after the consumption of one standard eight-ounce glass of milk. These symptoms may be reduced by drinking milk with a lower lactose content or by taking the milk with a meal.

Americans, in recent years, have complained bitterly about the rising cost of gasoline, which now costs more than a dollar a gallon in most parts of the country. When the lactase-deficient individual buys whole milk he is paying fifty cents or more for a quart of intestinal gas!

Studies have suggested that some of the nutritional benefits of milk may be lost when a lactase-deficient individual consumes milk. Not only does this person fail to receive the calories normally supplied by the undigested carbohydrates; resultant diarrhea may lead to loss of protein as well.

Bellyaches in children are quite common. It has been estimated that as many as one child in ten may experience the syndrome termed "recurrent abdominal pain of childhood." It is usually seen in children of school age; occurs over a period of months; is often worse in the mornings; and, in almost all instances, no evidence of disease can be found. Two studies were conducted in groups of children with "recurrent abdominal pain of childhood," one study performed in Boston and the other in San Francisco, came to a similar conclusion. The conclusion was that about one-third of such children had their symptoms on the basis of lactose intolerance. The simple solution was to remove all milk and milk-containing foods from the diet and watch for signs of improvement.

allergy to milk protein

Chapter 3

Don't Cry Over Spilt Milk

Brian Gordon was now two and a half years old and Mrs. Gordon had just about given up hope that he would ever be completely well. It all started around the age of six months when Brian began to have diarrhea. He soon became pale. Eventually he developed swelling of his hands and feet and his abdomen became bloated. Mrs. Gordon took Brian to several doctors in her small suburb. Many tests were performed but no satisfactory answers resulted. Brian's diet was changed from one formula to another but nothing seemed to help for any length of time. Brian was found to have iron-deficiency anemia but treatment with iron for months on end produced no improvement.

In desperation, Mrs. Gordon took Brian to a large medical center in hopes that somebody might be able to figure out what was wrong with her son. In just four days he was almost completely cured! Brian was found to be extremely sensitive to the protein in cow milk. As soon as Brian's diet was changed to exclude all protein derived from cows he immediately lost his swelling, his diarrhea stopped, and his blood count began to return to normal. Mrs. Gordon had tried Brian on a cow milk free diet in the past but it hadn't worked. Brian was so sensitive to the cow milk protein that *all* traces of it had to be removed from his diet. (There had been cow milk in the cookies Brian ate; in the custards he had for dessert; and in the beef he enjoyed several times a week.)

Although Brian's problem was extreme, allergy to cow milk is far more common than is generally appreciated. Dr. Joyce Gryboski, who directs the Pediatric Gastrointestinal Clinic at Yale University School of Medicine, states that they see at least one child a week who is referred for evaluation of chronic diarrhea and proves to have nothing more than an allergy to cow milk. This allergy may take many forms. Gastrointestinal disturbance is just one of the man ways that the allergy may make itself known. The most common form is believed by many to be chronic diarrhea. The stools range in consistency from several bothersome, soft, semiformed stools to numerous, watery explosive stools. Mucus is frequent and some stools contain obvious traces of bright red blood.

The symptoms usually begin shortly after a child begins to take whole cow milk but may also be observed in children who drink commercial formulas that include cows-milk protein. Those with mild symptoms grow well, but those with severe diarrhea are retarded in their weight gain. The diarrhea impairs the infant's ability to retain nutrients from his feedings. In addition, the changes produced in the gastrointestinal tract by the allergic reaction result in seepage of the child's own blood into the gut. This *edema*

loss of plasma and red cells leads to a lowering of the infant's blood protein level and to the development of anemia. The lowering of serum proteins, if profound, results in swelling of the abdomen, hands, and feet.

Most infants with this condition respond promptly to the elimination of cow milk from the diet. All symptoms may disappear within two days. Many of these infants may eventually develop the capacity to tolerate cow milk but this rarely occurs before the age of two. In some instances a child may be at least five years old before it is safe to feed him foods containing cow milk protein.

A less dramatic form of gastrointestinal sensitivity to cow milk is also being recognized with increasing frequency. This form of sensitivity rarely produces dramatic symptoms but results in slow and steady bleeding. Infants with this form of milk sensitivity may lose 1 to 5 milliliters of blood per day in their stool. Eventually they become anemic from the steady hemorrhage. The volumes of blood lost each day are too small for detection by simple visual examination. The stools appear to be of normal color and the blood can only be detected by chemical tests.

It is estimated that half the iron-deficiency in infants in the United States is primarily a result of this form of cow milk induced gastrointestinal bleeding. This is a staggering figure when one realizes that approximately 15 to 20 percent of all children under the age of two in this country suffer from iron-deficiency anemia.

scandal

In this condition, too, when cow milk is removed from the diet the bleeding ceases and treatment with iron medication corrects the anemia. If iron therapy is instituted while the child continues to drink cow milk, the blood loss goes on and offsets the benefits normally derived from the iron-containing medication.

The drinking of large quantities of cow milk has long been recognized to produce iron-deficiency anemia in infants. It has been assumed that the anemia was solely the result of the child not getting enough iron in his diet. Cow milk contains less than 1 milligram of iron per quart. Very little of this iron is absorbed from the intestinal tract because other constituents of the milk bind the iron and make it difficult for it to be taken up from the bowel into the blood. It has been estimated that an infant of one year of age would have to drink twenty-four quarts of milk per day to meet his iron requirements!

Many infants drink from one to two quarts of milk per day. This tends to satisfy their hunger and they are left with very little appetite for the necessary iron-containing foods. It would now appear that the consumption of cow milk by infants produces iron deficiency in two ways—it provides very little dietary iron and at the same time produces iron loss by inducing gastrointestinal bleeding.

The resultant iron-deficiency anemia makes the child irritable, apathetic, and inattentive. The infant cries a great deal, the mother gives a bottle of milk to soothe him, and the condition continues to get worse.

The recognition that excessive milk intake is often associated with iron deficiency has led to the description of "blue bottle syndrome." This syndrome is characterized by the toddler who is always walking around with a bottle in his hand. The bottle is filled with milk from which the child intermittently sucks. In the pre-plastic days it was unusual to see children drinking from bottles much after the first year of life. The infant, once he was up and around, would start dropping bottles. The glass bottles would break and after the infant broke a few bottles the mother would generally decide that it was time for her child to begin drinking from a cup. Now that the indestructible plastic bottle is available the economic pressure to institute cup drinking has been eliminated and it is not uncommon to see three- and even four-year-olds with bottles. These "milkaholics" are usually iron-deficient. Although plastic bottles do come in a variety of colors, the blue bottle appears to be the most popular among mothers and children; hence the term "blue bottle syndrome."

We have digressed from our theme of cow milk protein and cow milk allergy. Just how common is it and what are the symptoms, in addition to those that involve the gastrointestinal tract?

The incidence of allergy to cow milk has been variously estimated to range from as low as 0.3 percent of infants to as high as 25 percent. Obviously the criteria employed by physicians who make this diagnosis must be carefully examined in order to interpret their conclusions.

One of the most recent and most careful analyses of the problem of cow milk allergy was performed by Dr. J. W. Gerrard and associates in Saskatoon, Canada.

Dr. Gerrard and his colleagues personally supervised the care of 787 babies, consecutively admitted to their practice, in an attempt to determine the frequency of whole cow milk allergy. Infants were followed from birth. No attempt was made to persuade a mother to select one formula rather than another. A record was kept of the ages at which new foods were offered to the babies for the first time.

A baby with one or more of the following symptoms was considered a candidate for cow milk allergy and then studied further: (1) persistent or recurrent nasal congestion; attacks of asthma or chest infections; (2) persistent or recurrent skin rash; (3) vomiting or diarrhea (persistent or recurrent) for which no other explanation was present.

When a baby was thought to have an allergy to whole cow milk, he was taken off his cow milk formula and offered a formula prepared from soybeans instead. If his symptoms disappeared he was then again put on cow milk. If his symptoms returned he was again taken off milk and all other dairy products. When his symptoms subsided he was again "challenged" with milk and dairy products. Only if his symptoms returned on a second occasion was he considered allergic to cow milk.

Of the 787 babies studies, 59 were found to be allergic to cow milk—an overall incidence of 7.5 percent.

Symptoms seen most frequently in babies who are identified as allergic to cow milk included diarrhea, repeated vomiting, eczema, recurrent attacks of nasal congestion, and recurrent bronchitis.

A careful review of the mothers' diaries revealed that 25 percent of infants showed the first signs of their cow milk allergy within three days of being given a formula derived from cow milk and that almost half the children showed signs of their allergic problems within one week of starting such feedings.

The earlier in the child's life that he was fed cow milk, the more likely he was to develop allergic symptoms. Although the overall incidence of allergy to cow milk in children under one year of age was 7.5 percent, fully one in every four children who was fed cow milk before three months of age showed some signs of allergy.

Children who were allergic to cow milk saw their doctors much more frequently than the non-allergic children and required hospitalization on more occasions than the non-allergic child.

Dr. Gerrard and his colleagues also noted that allergy to cow milk was much more likely to develop in children whose parents or brothers and sisters had other allergic diseases. This was particularly true in the infants of parents who had had hay fever or asthma.

It would appear from these studies that the feeding of cow milk to human infants can produce disease and that the earlier the human infant is exposed to milk from another species, the more likely he is to show signs of intolerance. Studies of this type as well as the evidence that cow milk can produce gastrointestinal bleeding in young infants lends further support to the old adage, "Cow's milk is for cows."

And even more serious complication of cow milk has been described by a group of investigators from the University of Colorado and the University of Miami Schools of Medicine. Working together they have been able to identify a number of children ten to thirteen years old who had a troublesome form of persistent kidney disease known as nephrosis. Nephrosis is a disorder in which excess amounts of protein are lost from a damaged kidney. This continued loss of protein into the urine produces a lowering of the blood-protein level; and eventually results in pronounced fluid accumulation in the child. Children may have swollen hands and feet as well as fluid in their abdomen. Some children may go on to permanent renal disease and die.

Most children with nephrosis respond quite nicely to a variety of drugs. The drug that is most useful is derived from the adrenal gland and is a form of cortisone. But the children studied by the doctors in Colorado and Miami were patients who did not appear to benefit from cortisone. These physicians suspected that the children might be allergic to a variety of foods.

Much to their surprise and gratification, they found that when milk was removed from the diet these children promptly stopped losing protein in their urine and showed signs of marked improvement. When milk was added to the diets, within one to three days the urinary excretion of protein markedly increased. These investigators concluded that sensitivity to milk and other foods may play a major role in producing relapse in some children with nephrosis.

Other physicians noted additional relationships between cow milk and disease in children. Dr. J. Dan Baggett, a practicing pediatrician in Alabama, has been interested for a number of years in the possible harmful effects of cow milk. Here are portions of a letter written by Dr Baggett describing his experiences:

> When I opened my practice here in Montgomery, Alabama, in 1960, I was aware of a causal relationship between cow milk protein in the diet and infantile eczema. I also knew that many of these eczematoid children became asthmatics later on unless their eczema could be cleared early by dietary manipulation. This prompted me to begin a system of dietary prophylaxis against allergic disease among the newborns in my care. Only strained foods containing no milk, wheat, egg, or citrus were allowed through age nine months.
>
> When my babies developed eczema, they were promptly switched to a soy formula and although most of these did well, a few of them

would clear, only to eventually develop eczema from the soy. Usually, there were further alternatives available, allowing me to raise them without eczema.

Gradually I became aware of the demonstrable relationship of food items in the causation of several respiratory and gastrointestinal disorders.

In 1964, I learned of the experiences of Dr. William Deamer of San Francisco. He had pointed out the frequency of milk protein's causal relationship to musculoskeletal pain in children and especially the so-called "growing pains."

Since that time, I have had several children with what appeared to be early rheumatoid arthritis relieved and returned to good health by little more than reassurance and careful dietary manipulation.

About six years ago, I began systematically persuading every patient of mine to delete all cow milk products from their diets. In general, they cooperate much better than I had earlier anticipated except for the pre-teenagers and teenagers.

My patients are all given a list of "legal" breads, crackers, cake mixes, and cookies containing no casein, caseinate, whey, or milk solids. They are allowed small amounts of butter (contains 2 percent whey) and a 100 percent corn-oil margarine. Corn oil and safflower oil are recommended for cooking. They are, in addition, given a modification of Dr. W.L. Deamer's milk-protein avoidance list to assist them in their shopping habits.

During the years 1963 through 1967, I referred an average of four appendectomy cases per year. During the past five and a half years, I have referred only two patients for appendectomy, the last one being three years ago. Both of these children were professed milk guzzlers.

I do not have a single patient with active asthma. In fact, I have nearly forgotten how to prescribe for them.

Perhaps the most significant thing I have learned is that Group A beta-hemolytic streptococcus germ will not, under ordinary circumstances, establish an infection in a child kept on an absolutely no-milk-protein dietary regimen. I have been aware of this for the past two and a half years and, so far, there have been no exceptions. Any time a patient of mine is found to have streptococcal pharyngitis or pyoderma, we can establish by history that he has ingested milk protein within five days prior to onset of symptoms or signs bringing him to the office.

I now admit an average of 12-14 patients per year to the hospital. Their average hospital stay is three days. Between 1963 and 1967, I admitted an average of 100+ patients to the hospital per year. Their average hospital stay was five days.

Breast fed is best fed and cow milk is the ideal food for the newly born and rapidly growing calf.

My nursing mothers are advised to eat eggs, if tolerated, and dark green leafy vegetables and to take prenatal vitamins and bone-meal tablets for an abundance of calcium. They are advised to eschew all cow milk protein, chocolate, cola drinks, peanuts, and raw onion, and to eat anything else they want that doesn't upset their nursing baby. Such a wonderful experience is in store for them when they do it "right."

The observation relating streptococcal disease to milk protein in the diet can be verified by most any pediatrician with time and patience to test it. It is often helpful to ask the child first whether he has had milk, ice cream, or cheese in his diet within the week prior to the office visit where strep is suspected. This cuts down on the embarrassment of having the child volunteer information contrary to the parent's story.

As human beings we show great variability in what we are able to tolerate in what we eat. For many of us it is quite apparent that cow milk will produce disease. Since the human infant was never supposed to drink cow milk in the first place, it is not surprising that they appear most vulnerable. And since no animal drinks milk after he's weaned, it is not surprising that the drinking of cow milk after one to two years of age will also produce disease. What is surprising is how frequently cow milk does produce disturbances and how long it has taken for the medical profession to recognize this factor.

Allergies to Milk was published in 1980. The authors of this book which is a comprehensive text and extensive catalogue of what we presently know about this subject, are Sami Bahna and Douglas Heiner. For the reader wishing to pursue the current scientific foundation for the immunologic basis of milk allergy the book by Doctors Bahna and Heiner can be highly recommended. In the first chapter of the book they begin with the following:

"Until recently, allergy to cow's milk was a controversial subject toward which many physicians had differing attitudes. Some

textbooks of pediatrics either avoid mentioning cow's milk allergy or only lightly refer to its relation to gastrointestinal symptoms. A few clinicians do not believe the condition exists and thus are understandably reluctant to diagnose it. On the other hand, there are those, particularly among pediatricians, and to a lesser extent among general practitioners, who over-zealously label infants "milk-sensitive" and who are inclined to recommend discontinuing the use of cow's milk whenever an infant has a gastrointestinal upset, respiratory symptoms, or a skin rash. Among the reasons for such divergent attitudes are (1) the variety of symptoms caused by cow's milk allergy, many of which may also occur as manifestations of other morbid conditions, and (2) the lack of a reliable single practical laboratory test. Public awareness of cow's milk allergy, though increasing, is still marginal. Parents frequently are incredulous that milk could cause the symptoms their infant is exhibiting. The prevailing attitude is that cow's milk is not only a desirable food, but the ideal food and an essential element of the child's diet."

Chapter 4

Can Fat Be Fatal?

Organizations such as the American Heart Association have strongly urged that the consumption of milk and other dairy products be reduced by Americans of all ages—and for good reason. Diseases of the heart and major blood vessels will kill about one million Americans this year. These diseases are responsible for one out of two deaths that occur in this country. Of this million deaths, approximately two-thirds will be due to heart attacks. Even more chilling is the fact that somewhere between 150,000 and 200,000 deaths due to heart attacks will occur in individuals under sixty-five years of age—mostly men in their productive years of life.

We have done very little to change these statistics. Everyone knows that an infant born in 1977 can expect to live far longer than one born in 1900. The infant born in 1900 could look forward to a life of fifty years while the infant born today can reasonably expect to live an average of seventy-two years. Unexpressed in these numbers is the fact that the increased life expectancy is a result of the elimination of many diseases that killed people during infancy and childhood. The eradication of many infectious diseases with vaccines; better care of newborns; and the general improvement of nutrition are largely responsible for these gains.

When you reached age forty-five in 1900, you had a reasonable prospect of living to age seventy; today the forty-five-year-old person can expect to live to age seventy-six. A gain of only six years in life expectancy in the last seventy-five years. Why? Because we have yet to significantly reduce the death rate from atherosclerosis.

Atherosclerosis, one of the group of blood-vessel diseases called arteriosclerosis, is a disorder characterized by thick, irregular deposits on the inner lining of arteries. These "plaques" restrict blood flow through the artery and thus compromise the oxygen supply to the organ supplied by the artery. These roughened spots can break loose, or cause rupture of the artery by weakening the blood vessel's wall or, most importantly, provide a location for the formation of a blood clot. A blood clot in an artery will completely prevent blood flow.

This process of vessel obstruction, as a result of atherosclerosis, can occur in any artery of the body, but it is most common in the large and middle-sized arteries supplying the brain, kidneys, legs, and heart. When blood circulation is obstructed in the brain, a "stroke" results; when the process occurs in the heart it is termed a "heart attack" or coronary artery occlusion. The occlusion of one of the three coronary arteries results in death of the heart muscle which the vessel normally supplies. Muscle or tissue death is called "infarction; hence the phrase "myocardial infarction" to signify the consequences of impaired blood supply to the heart.

What are the cause of atherosclerosis? Until the 1950's, most people believed that hardening of the arteries was just a normal accompaniment of aging. The findings uncovered during the Korean War changed all that. Autopsies performed on our young soldiers, most of them in their late teens or early twenties, revealed that almost eighty percent already have evidence of atherosclerosis. Subsequent studies demonstrated that early signs of atherosclerosis may be present even in children two or three years of age!

The arterial-vessel plaque deposition is a slow process that generally unfolds over twenty to forty years. The plaques are rich in fat—most notably cholesterol. Most Americans, by the time they reach age fifty, have evidence of severe atherosclerosis. Is this an inevitable process or can it be prevented or retarded?

The primary event that causes injury to the lining of the artery which then becomes the site for buildup of the atherosclerotic plaque is still unknown. What has been recognized, however, is that the disease occurs with increased frequency and severity when certain risk factors are present.

These risk factors include high blood cholesterol, the ratio of high density lipoprotein (HDL) to low density lipoprotein (LDL) in the serum, high blood pressure, diabetes, cigarette smoking, sedentary living, certain personality traits, and family history of heart attacks and strokes. The more risk factors present, the greater a person's chances of suffering the ravages of atherosclerosis at any age. The presence of an increased serum concentration of high density lipoprotein appears to reduce the risk of heart attacks for any given serum cholesterol level.

The concept of "risk factors" has grown out of studies supported by the National Institutes of Health in Framingham, Massachusetts. This factory town outside Boston has a population of some 28,000 and represents an accurate cross-section of the United States in terms of economic status and ethnic mix. In 1949, some 5,000 healthy men and women between the ages of thirty and fifty-nine were selected for careful study. Every other year these individuals underwent careful physical exams and laboratory tests. Over the years, about a thousand of these residents of Framingham had died. The factors contributing to their deaths have helped provide scientists with the data used to formulate the concept of "risk factors."

Because so many factors predispose to the development of atherosclerosis it has been hard to identify any one alone as most important. While there is no unanimity of opinion, most investigators believe that a high blood cholesterol level is the most important risk factor—particularly when it occurs in association with a genetic or inherited predisposition to the disease.

Diet is an important factor in determining serum cholesterol levels. Cholesterol in the plasma and body tissues is derived from two sources: the foods we eat and the cholesterol that we produce in the liver and intestines. The typical adult in this country consumes a diet containing 600 to 800 milligrams per day, which is much higher than in most other part of the world. This cholesterol comes from food products of animal origin such as egg yolks, dairy fats, and meat. The more you eat, the more you absorb into your system. In addition, 500 to 1,000 milligrams of cholesterol are produced each day by the body. This production goes on almost independent of the amount consumed in the diet.

Two substances in the diet appear to control the plasma level of cholesterol: the cholesterol and the saturated fat that you eat. Saturated fats are usually solid at room temperature. Foods such as butter, cheese, cream, beef, pork, lamb, and chocolate are rich in saturated fats. The ingestion of saturated fats makes serum cholesterol levels rise. Unsaturated fats are usually liquids at room temperature. Corn oil, cottonseed oil, safflower oil, and other vegetable oils are rich in unsaturated fats. The ingestion of unsaturated fats makes serum cholesterol levels fall.

The first evidence of a relationship between diet and atherosclerosis was provided between 1910 and 1920 by a Russian investigator, Nikolai Anitschov. Rabbits fed a diet rich in fat and cholesterol quickly developed atherosclerosis. Since that time, many animal studies have produced atherosclerosis by means of diets rich in cholesterol.

It is obviously far more difficult to conduct similar experiments in man. Indirect evidence has been employed to demonstrate a link between diet, cholesterol, and heart disease and stroke. The Framingham project indicated that men with a blood cholesterol level of 240 milligrams had three times as many heart attacks as men with blood cholesterol levels of less than 200 milligrams percent.

Surveys of world populations have shown a direct statistical relationship between blood cholesterol levels and the incidence of heart attacks. In general, throughout the world there is a direct relationship between serum cholesterol levels, atherosclerosis, and the consumption of dairy products and meats.

There are about 35 grams of fat in a quart of milk. About 60 percent of the fat of milk is in the saturated form. If you drink one quart of whole milk per day you will have consumed over one-third of your daily quota of fat as recommended by both the American Heart Association and the White House panel on Food, Nutrition, and Health. Drinking that much milk allows very little flexibility in the choice of other fat-containing foods in the daily diet. In addition, the consumption of milk fat–rich in saturates–provides almost all the presumed safe amount of this component as well.

Simple dietary changes can reduce the mortality from heart attacks. The most convincing evidence comes from a study conducted in Finland in two large hospitals with stable patient populations. From 1959 to 1965, patients in Hospital N were provided with a cholesterol-lowering diet while patients in Hospital K were fed normal institutional fare. In 1965, the diets were reversed. The experimental diet differed from the usual diet in only two major respects: whole cow milk was replaced by a "filled milk"—an emulsion of soybean oil in skimmed milk; and a "soft" margarine, rich in polyunsaturated fat, was substituted for butter or ordinary margarine.

The experimental diet produced an average reduction in serum cholesterol levels of close to 20 percent. More importantly, it reduced by over half the death rate from coronary artery disease among the males in the study. Although other studies have also suggested the same beneficial effects from dietary modification, this particular study is most impressive in view of the minor dietary manipulations require to produce such a large desirable effect.

The American dairy industry is also concerned that the fat in milk may be harmful. This is reflected by the large-scale production of skimmed milk and low-fat milk. Even "ice milk" has been produced as a substitute for ice cream.

Prudent diets can reduce cholesterol levels and probably reduce the death rate from heart disease. Recent calculations suggest that for middle-aged men with normal blood pressure who do not smoke, adoption of a prudent diet alone could save six of every hundred of them from heart attacks. The benefits are even greater if other risk factors are already present. If the men were smokers who already had evidence of heart enlargement, commencing a diet designed to lower blood cholesterol levels would help twenty-nine per hundred to escape heart attacks.

Pediatricians have also been alerted to the important role they must play in the prevention of atherosclerosis. Authorities recommend that all children in families in which there is a parent or grandparent with a history of a heart attack before age fifty be screened for evidence of disturbance in the way the body transports and regulates fat. Blood samples should be obtained by the age of one year in children from such families. The blood levels of cholesterol and triglycerides should be measured. If either of these is elevated, then further studies should be conducted to determine if a genetic abnormality in the fat-transport proteins of the blood is present. Different types of abnormalities require different forms of dietary management. Some may require drug treatment as well.

The most common of these inherited abnormalities in fat transport is termed Type II hyperlipoproteinemia. It affects about one in every 200 members of the population. It has been estimated that about 5 percent of males with this trait will develop evidence of heart disease by the time they are thirty years of age, about 50 percent will have heart disease by age fifty, and 85 percent by age sixty. In this, the most common form of inherited disturbance, the recommended diet severely limits the intake of cholesterol by reducing consumption of eggs, fatty meats, shellfish, *and* dairy products. Such diets should be instituted around one year of age.

The consumption of cow milk from an early age may have life-long consequences. Changes that are believed to represent the forerunners of atherosclerosis have been observed in the coronary vessels of infants and children. One pathologist has reviewed the heart vessels of over 1,500 children and adolescents who had died as a result of accidents. Deaths were a result of auto injuries, drownings, gunshot wounds, and related traumas. These children and adolescents had not died as a result of disease, yet many of them showed signs of diseased arteries in the heart.

When an attempt was made to unravel the factors responsible for the fact that some of these children and adolescents had normal blood vessels and others did not, the single feature that most clearly distinguished the two groups was their early feeding histories. The majority of children with normal blood vessels had been breast-fed; the majority of children with diseased vessels had been fed cow milk or cow milk based formulas. It is therefore reasonable to conclude that the differences between human milk and cow milk were responsible for the early changes in the coronary arteries.

All the findings that link diet to atherosclerosis underscore the belief that cow milk was not designed for human consumption. The life-long consumption of milk is not practiced by any species of mammal except the human. Atherosclerosis is unknown among other mammals. It can only be produced by the feeding of human-type diets—diets rich in fat and cholesterol. In February of 1977 the United States Senate Select Committee on Nutrition and Human Needs released a document entitled, "Dietary Goals for the United States." In this report, one of the recommendations was that Americans reduce their intake of fat and suggested that efforts be made to reduce the intake of milk and other dairy products. Many organizations, including quite naturally the National Dairy Council, challenged the recommendations.

In 1982 came another salvo. The National Research Council issued a report entitled, *Diet, Nutrition and Cancer*. This report was a milestone in that it represented the first time any official body had suggested that the risk of cancer could be reduced by dietary changes. Among the recommendations was that the proportion of calories provided by fats should be reduced from 40 percent to 30 percent in the average American diet. The report states, "Of all the dietary compounds studied the combined epidemiological and experimental evidence is most suggestive for a causal relationship between fat intake and the occurrence of cancer"—particularly cancers of the colon, breast and prostate.

The diet designed to help reduce the incidence of heart disease may also reduce the risk of cancer. The American Heart Association called it a "prudent diet." No guarantees, no money back offers. It does appear, however, that it would be prudent to reduce fat intake if it might prevent both heart disease and cancer.

One quart of whole milk per day adds 35 grams of fat to your diet. This 35 grams represents about one-half of all the fat you should consume in one day if you are the average 150 pound man. Is that the way you wish to spend your fat allotment?

Even more exciting is the evidence that is accumulating that suggests that eating less of the proper foods may actually extend the normal life span. In the June 8, 1982, edition of *The New York Times*, Jane *caloric restriction*

Brody, in an article titled, "Eating Less May Be The Key to Living Beyond 100 Years" summarizes the animal data that suggests that longevity can be increased by consuming a diet containing all the proper nutrients, but a third less calories than are needed to maintain a "normal" body weight. The benefits of under-nutrition can be gained even when such a diet is instituted in middle age. All the evidence to date has come from animal studies but there is every reason to believe that they are applicable to humans.

Reduce your fat intake, reduce your caloric intake—you may find yourself eating for a much longer time than you thought possible.

During the first year of life the infant should be fed human milk or a commercial preparation that resembles human milk as closely as possible. A variety of milks are now available for that purpose. After one to two years of age, the time of normal weaning, milk should be removed from the diet.

Chapter 5

The Alternatives—Two Sides To The Story

If cow milk is eliminated from the diet, what are the alternatives? Clearly the alternatives to drinking cow milk are different for infants and children than they are for adults. In this chapter we will begin to examine the alternatives for infants. For the newborn infant there are two obvious alternatives—the right and left breast of the healthy mother. Although commercial infant formulas derived from cow milk or soy proteins are adequate to support the growth of most infants, human milk is the ideal food for virtually all infants.

Commercial infant formulas have been gradually modified over the thirty years since their introduction and now tend to approximate human milk in their content of fat, protein, and carbohydrate. But the commercial formulas have not been able to duplicate human milk in the degree of protection it affords against infections.

Breast milk, and most particularly colostrum the milk secreted by the human breast during the first days after the birth of an infant, is rich in substances that confer immunity on the baby during the period of life when he is most susceptible to life-threatening infections. Breast milk is rich in antibodies. These proteins are necessary for the body's defense against infection by bacteria and viruses.

There is much evidence to support the conviction that infants fed on human milk are less prone to illness than those who aren't. A study of over twenty thousand infants conducted in Chicago as far back as the 1930s illustrates this point.

Remember that this study was conducted long before antibiotics were available for bacterial infections. Any increase in illness or mortality could therefore be presumed to be a result of harmful products in the cow milk or the absence of protective factors in the human milk. In this study, one group of infants was breast-fed for at least the first nine months of age; a second group was partially breast-fed; and a third group was raised on a diluted, boiled cow milk with added sugar. All infants were given orange juice starting at one month of age and cod-liver oil at six weeks. Cereal was added to the diet at five months of age and a vegetable when the infants were six months old.

What happened? The overall death rate for the babies raised on human milk was 1.5 per 1,000 infants while the death rate in the babies fed cow milk was 84.7 per 1,000 infants during the first nine months of life. The death rate from gastrointestinal infections was forty times higher in the non-breast-fed infants, while the death rate from respiratory infection was 120 times higher.

An earlier analysis involving infants in eight American cities showed similar results. Infants fed on cow milk had a twenty times greater chance of dying during the first six months of life.

Today, in the United States it would be difficult to demonstrate that infants fed on human milk have a better chance of survival. Antibiotics and better means of supporting infants during life-threatening illnesses reduce the mortality in infants who do not receive human milk. In areas of the world that have less well-developed medical-care systems, the death rate in babies not receiving human milk is still unacceptably high.

For example, during the first six months of life in Chile, the mortality rates for bottle-fed infants is twice as high as in infants who are exclusively breast-fed. Breast-fed babies who received supplements of cow milk do no better than infants who only receive cow milk. This suggests that if a baby is to benefit from breast milk he must receive breast milk alone.

The study in Chile also demonstrated that as income rose, mothers tended to switch from breast feeding to bottle feeding. This switch accounted for the striking finding that mortality rates for infants was higher in the families with better incomes.

The protective value of breast feeding has also been demonstrated in a series of studies in Guatemala. Observations were made on a group of breast-fed infants in an isolated community where standards of hygiene were poor and the sanitation system was primitive. Samples of the infants' stools were taken at weekly intervals for bacterial cultures. While the infants were exclusively breast-fed, their stools contained only a strain of harmless bacterium-Lactobacillus. None of the infants experienced attacks of gastroenteritis. However, gastroenteritis was common in the infants who were artificially fed.

As soon as mothers began to wean their infants, the type of bacteria in the stool abruptly changed. The stools now contained the bacterial species *E. coli*. This species is known to produce a variety of infections–in the central nervous system, lungs, kidneys, and bloodstream–of infants. This bacterium first establishes residence in the intestinal tract and from there spreads to other parts of the body when the host's resistance is altered. Since the feeding of human milk–and human milk along–prevents the growth of *E. coli*, this form of infection is virtually unknown in the exclusively breast-fed infant.

Outbreaks of gastroenteritis in nurseries can be halted by the feeding of human milk. Such epidemics have been brought under control with human milk after all other efforts have failed. A careful analysis of an epidemic in a nursery in Belgrade, Yugoslavia, is most illuminating. During a period of six months, all infants–a total of 1,008–admitted to the nursery were surveyed. In this period, 883 babies were put to the breast–none developed gastroenteritis and none had *E. coli* in their stool cultures. The other 125 infants received boiled human milk. In this group sixteen developed gastroenteritis and all had *E. coli* in their stools. After this experience all infants received fresh human milk, and within two months *E. coli* was gone from the nursery.

The protective benefits of mother's milk are well recognized by farmers. When a calf or piglet does not receive milk from the cow or sow during the first twenty-four hours of life, the animals frequently develop gastrointestinal infections and die.

The milk of each species appears to have been specifically designed to protect the young of that species.

Cross-feeding does not work. Heating, sterilization, or modification of the milk in any way destroys the protection.

In virtually every mammal that has been studied to date exclusive milk drinking is practiced until the animal has approximately tripled its birth weight. This may be as long as three years for an elephant or as short as three weeks for a guinea pig. If humans were to follow this rule of nature, exclusive breast feeding would have to continue until about one year of age.

Certainly most infants in Western societies can grow well on commercial infant formulas (see next chapter). The incidence of infections does not appear to be unacceptably high but the immunologic advantage does rest with the infant who is fed on human milk.

Unfortunately, customs in well-developed countries are often imitated in more primitive countries. The results can be disastrous. Growing numbers of women in developing countries are abandoning breast feeding. In Chile, for example, the rate of breast feeding has fallen from 95 percent to 6 percent within twenty years. The duration of breast feeding has fallen from an average of a little over one year to an average of two months.

Among the factors responsible for this switch to commercial formulas are an increasing trend for women to work; the desire on the part of lower-class women to imitate women in the local upper classes as well as in the more highly industrialized Western societies; the availability of powdered milk from international health agencies; and the vigorous and largely irresponsible promotion of commercial formulas by manufacturers.

Some manufacturers have employed the strategy of creating a "need" where none really existed. When women in South American or African countries see a fat, healthy baby drinking from a bottle on a poster in their health clinic they interpret it as an endorsement of the product. Billboards, magazine advertising, and other subtle marketing techniques are employed to convince the prospective mother that she should feed her infant in the modern way.

In most of the poor countries the commercial infant formulas are sold in powdered form. The reconstitution of this powder into a safe infant feed requires a measuring device, a source of pure water, and clean (preferably sterile), bottles and nipples. For women living in poverty—who usually do not have a source of refrigeration, easy access to pure water, common measuring devices, and an ability to read instruction, the infant formula is not a convenience but a harmful inconvenience.

Leah Marguiles in an article entitled "Baby Formula Abroad: Exporting Infant Malnutrition" clearly summarizes this problem. She writes:

> *In the past few years there has been documentation of insidious marketing and promotional techniques employed by companies aggressively competing to increase their share in a fast-expanding and, thus far, unsaturated market. Recent figures from Jamaica reveal that 90 percent of Kingston mothers started bottle feeding before six months, with 14 percent of this group saying that they were encouraged to do so by a commercial "milk nurse." They were approached through both hospitals and postnatal clinics.*
>
> *This usual practice–implemented by what the American companies describe as their*

"mothercraft personnel"–is but one part of the high-pressure campaign operating within the health-care services of the countries involved. Companies also advertise on radio, billboards, and occasionally on TV. In some cases milk nurses are hired to visit neighborhoods and may even be paid on a commission basis. Most companies, however, employ nurses on their regular payrolls to promote the products through doctors, hospitals, and maternity and postnatal clinics: *"ninety-five percent of the [Nigerian] mothers who combined breast and bottle feeding believed they had been advised to do so by personnel, mainly midwives or nurses. Milk company personnel who give talks on feeding appear to be identified as hospital and clinic staff."*

A Nestle's spokesman attempted to whitewash the practice by saying that *"the nurse is the counterpart of what in the pharmaceutical industry is the detail man who visits doctors and health centers and informs them about their products."* This analogy, however, is false. Doctors are experts in a position to make informed choices. Imagine the reaction of a third world mother in her home, or a group of mothers in a clinic or hospital attending a class, to a woman in a crisp nurse's uniform. The woman may or may not be a nurse. She begins her speech, tactfully enough, by reassuring them that *"breast is best,"* but she ends by extolling the virtues of her company's product over the natural method. By capitalizing on the respect given a nurse the technique implies a connection between the health-care profession and the commercial product. This *"mothercraft"* *employee embodies the dynamics and vitality necessary for the growth of markets, not care for the growth of infants....* [*]

The marketing techniques that Marguiles criticizes have been very successful. They have also been very destructive. What has happened in Chile is a sad example of this success. In 1973 three times as many deaths occurred among infants who were bottle-fed before three months of age than among wholly breast-fed infants.

Marguiles goes on to cite the reasons for the increased death rate among the bottle-fed infants. Responsible factors include such things as contaminated water supplies, lack of facilities for boiling of water and inability to read instructions necessary for the preparation of the formula.

The author goes on to state:

Malnutrition is another common result and has been described as "commerciogenic malnutrition." This is not meant to imply that the manufacturers are solely responsible but simply that this type of malnutrition has nothing directly to do with underdevelopment and lack of food resources. It results from practices and policies that are derived from pseudodevelopment and the commercialization process....

Since 1973 pressure has been applied to the companies most involved in selling commercial infant formulas to the poor countries of the world. A third-world group has published a pamphlet entitled

---

[*] Reprinted from the November 10, 1975 issue of Christianity and Crisis, © 1975 by Christianity and Crisis, Inc., 537 West 121 Street, New York 10027.

"Nestle's Kills Babies." Nestle's, in Switzerland, has filed a libel suit.

In England, attention to this problem was produced by Mike Muller in *The Baby Killer*. In this book he describes in detail the subtle abuses in infant feeding practices produced by the manufacturers of commercial formulas. In the United States, Consumers Union has also investigated the situation and concluded in *Hungry for Profits* that commercial interests were permitted to override the human concerns of the population.

Lives are being lost in these developing countries as a result of this commercialization of infant feeding practices. As distressing is the diversion of national resources in these already poor countries. In Kenya, for example, it is estimated that the decline in breast feeding of babies has required the expenditure of eleven and a half million dollars for human milk substitutes for infants. This represents two-thirds of the nation's entire health budget and is equal to one-fifth of all the economic aid this troubled nation currently receives. Human milk can be viewed as a national economic resource as well as a natural resource.

In 1981 the World Health Organization passed a resolution banning the promotion of infant formulas in developing countries and endorsed the concept that all infants should be breast-fed whenever possible.

A quiet revolution in infant feeding practices has taken place here in the United States during the past decade. In 1971 only 25 percent of infants were being breast-fed at the time of discharge from the hospital nursery—now the figure has risen to 58 percent. Even more striking has been the delay in the introduction of whole cow milk to the baby's diet. In 1971, 68 percent of infants were receiving cow milk or evaporated milk by the time they were 6 months of age. In 1981, the number of infants being fed in such a fashion has dropped to only 17 percent. The fact that breast feeding is the best way to feed all babies has been endorsed by the American Academy of Pediatrics, the American Pediatric Society, the Pediatric Research Society, and the Pediatric Ambulatory Association. Even the National Dairy Council now openly acknowledges that whole cow milk is not a suitable feed for infants during the first 6 months of life. Progress—yes. Perfection—no.

In the Western world children who are not breast-fed can be raised on commercial formulas. Raised more expensively, but nevertheless raised, employing sound nutritional principles. Ideally the infant should be exclusively fed human milk for the first year of life. If this is not possible, or desirable, then the infant should be fed a commercial formula for the first year. The infant should never receive cow milk in an unmodified form. After the first year of life the child requires no milk of any type. The child, like us adults, can thrive without cow milk ever crossing his lips.

Chapter 6

The Calcium Scare

"But doctor, what will happen to my teeth and bones if I stop drinking milk?"

That question, or some version of it, is the one most frequently asked when I suggest to people that milk be removed from the diet. Most Americans know that milk is rich in calcium. Most Americans know that you need lots of calcium to have strong bones and healthy teeth. Most Americans know these facts because the dairy industry told them so.

Most Americans also knew that Thomas E. Dewey was "sure" to become the thirty-fourth President of the United States (until, on Election Day, he didn't).

What most Americans don't know, and don't even stop to think about, is that the majority of the world's population takes in less than half the calcium we are told we need and yet, by and large, has strong bones and healthy teeth.

There are approximately 1,200 milligrams of calcium in a quart of milk. It is indeed one of the foods that is rich in calcium. The Food and Nutrition Board of the National Academy of Sciences recommends that adults have 800 milligrams of calcium in their diet each day. Other distinguished committees in their countries, drawing on the same research, have drawn different conclusions. For example, in the United Kingdom and Canada the recommended daily allowance is 500 milligrams per day and a range of only 400 to 500 milligrams per day has been recommended by the Food and Agriculture Division of the World Health Organization.

Why the difference of opinion? Establishing calcium requirements is an extremely complicated business. The amount of calcium in your diet is only one factor in determining how much calcium gets into your body. Many other things you eat may interfere with calcium absorption from the intestinal tract. These include the amount of phosphates, fiber, and protein in your diet. In addition, vitamin D and body hormones play an important role in increasing calcium absorption.

The lack of relationship between the calcium in your diet and the amount that ultimately gets into your blood and then to your bones and teeth is best illustrated by the comparisons that have been made between infants drinking human milk or cow milk. As I've said previously, cow milk contains 1,200 milligrams of calcium per quart; human milk has only 300 milligrams per quart. Yet, despite these differences, the infant receiving human milk *actually absorbs more calcium into his body*.

The reason has to do with the fact that cow milk is also rich in phosphorus. The ratio of calcium to phosphorus is somewhat greater than two to one. Phosphorus can combine with calcium in the intestinal tract and prevent the absorption of calcium. Many nutritionists believe that only foods with a calcium-to-phosphorus ratio of two to one or better should be used as a primary source of calcium.

Let us get back to the problems of calcium in adults. Studies have been performed in which the bone density or bone strength of various populations have been compared. Comparisons have been made between members of populations in which calcium intake is similar to that recommended in the United States and members of populations, primarily Africans, in which daily calcium, intake is less than half that recommended for Americans. The results indicate that there was no evidence of bone softness in those populations with a reduced calcium intake.

As more studies are performed it has become increasingly clear that we know very little about how much calcium humans really need to maintain good health. It is known that too much and too little calcium can be harmful. But how little is too little remains a mystery. African nations and blacks in this country, groups that consume far less calcium than most Caucasians, tend to have less softening of bone (osteoporosis) and in fact have bones of greater density. These findings have led Dr. Alexander Walker of the South African Institute for Medical Research to state, "There is no firm evidence that calcium deficiency exists in humans."

This may represent an extreme view, but an expert group from the World Health Organization has concluded that there is no convincing evidence that calcium intakes of less than 300 milligrams a day are harmful to the health. And 300 milligrams a day represents the calcium in one glass of cow milk.

A more timid conclusion, which nonetheless runs counter to popular belief, was reached by the Nutrition Committee of the American Academy of Pediatrics. This group stated: "From the viewpoint of calcium requirements alone, the amounts of milk recommended for daily consumption by children and adolescents (three or more glasses for children, four or more for adolescents) in both popular and official health statements could be above what is required for normal skeletal, dental, and general growth and development."

It is apparent that the human body can adjust to variations in the amount of calcium in the diet. When calcium is eaten in reduced quantities, apparently more is absorbed in an attempt to meet needs.

The average American gets 807 milligrams a day of calcium from drinking milk. The average Spaniard gets 308 milligrams a day from milk; the Brazilian 250 milligrams; the Taiwanese 13 milligrams; and the average citizen of Ghana gets 8 milligrams. These non-American people are neither toothless nor lying about immobilized because of repeated bone fractures.

Everybody does need some calcium. Fortunately, there are a variety of foods that are rich in this mineral. For example, 3 ounces of sardines, one ounce of Swiss cheese, one cup of cooked collards, one cup of turnips, or 4 ounces of flour, all provide more than 250 milligrams of calcium. More than 200 milligrams of calcium can be obtained from a cup oysters, a cup of cooked rhubarb, a cup of cottage cheese, or a 4 ounce serving of salmon; in addition, kidney beans, broccoli, soybeans, almonds, a variety of fish, and cassava are good sources of calcium.

"But, doctor, what will happen to my teeth and bones if I stop drinking milk?" Nothing. Nothing that wouldn't have happened anyway.

Chapter 7

Do You Really Want a Resumé of the Cow's Lunch?

"The quality of a number of the dairy products in this study was little short of deplorable" was the conclusion reached by the Consumers Union survey published in the January,

1974 issue of *Consumer Reports*. The article was aptly entitled, "Milk: Why Is the Quality So Low?"

Americans who regard milk as "the perfect food" rarely think about milk as a commercial product—with all the potential faults and hazards of everything else we buy at the store. The investigators from Consumers Union examined milk as a product and evaluated it for taste, bacterial contamination, and undesirable additives. Their findings should frighten even the milkaholics away from their local dairy bars.

Consumers Union sampled milk originating in processing plants in Iowa, Illinois, Kansas, Arkansas,
and Missouri. These five states produce about 11 percent of the nation's supply. The consultants tested at
least three samples from each of twenty-five brands.
First they judged the taste. Only 12 percent of all the
samples tested were found to be free of some defect
that compromised the taste of the product. Different
samples from the same brand varied so widely with
respect to taste that reliance on brand name as a
guide to milk became impossible. (Would you be satis-
fied if each bottle of Coca-Cola had a different taste?)

Over one-third of the milk samples contained flavors of the feed recently eaten by the cow. The taste of
wild garlic or wild onion will appear in milk within
hours after the cow has sampled them. Even worse; if
a cow merely inhales the odor of garlic, the flavor will
appear in the milk in a matter of minutes. Corn, oats,
rye, apple pomace, turnips, and bitterweed also will
convey their flavors to milk after being eaten by the
cow. Corn, oats, and rye are standard fodder for most
cows. All feedings should be withheld for several
hours before milking in order to reduce this type of
taste adulteration. When cows are fed right up until
milking, the milk you drink will be a "resumé of the
cow's lunch."

Many of the milks also tasted cooked. This was a
result of sloppy processing: the milks had been held at
a high temperature too long. Heating of milk is necessary to sterilize the product but when the temperature
is too high (or maintained too long) the results are
readily apparent to the palate. Do you remember the
last time you tasted boiled milk?

In addition to the traces of cow fodder and the
cooked taste, many of the milks also seemed flat or
oxidized. Oxidation may result from improper refrig-

eration or from the absorption into the milk of chemicals present in the container. Even worse, one of the whole-milk samples tasted soapy

So much for taste—what about sterility? Many of the samples failed this test as well.

Milk from a healthy cow will always contain some bacteria. These usually originate from fecal matter that has contaminated the cow's udder and teats. Dairy farmers recognize this hazard and generally cleanse the cow's udder both before and after milking. In addition, the milking machines are, or should be, continually cleaned. Once milk has been collected, it can be further contaminated by the microbes in the environment. Warm milk is an excellent culture medium for the growth of many of these bacteria. Prompt cooling of the milk will help retard the growth of potentially dangerous microorganisms.

Because it is recognized that it is impossible for milk to remain free of all contamination, it is heated (pasteurized) at the processing plant to destroy bacteria. This is designed to kill disease-producing organisms such as coliform bacteria and tuberculosis bacilli. The pasteurization process, by reducing the number of organisms in the milk, allows the milk to be stored longer. It also inactivates enzymes, normally present in milk, which may modify its flavor.

Since the drinking of unpasteurized milk was frequently responsible for epidemics, The U.S. Public Health Service developed standards to prevent such occurrences. The government regulation states that milk, after pasteurization, should contain no more than 20,000 bacteria per milliliter of milk and no more than ten organisms of the coliform species in each milliliter. (For those readers who don't normally deal in milliliters, there are 5 milliliters in a teaspoon and 30 milliliters in an ounce.)

Note that the government doesn't expect the milk to be sterile after pasteurization; it just wants the number of bacteria kept at a respectable minimum. Bacteria grow rapidly in milk which isn't appropriately refrigerated. At 40 degrees Fahrenheit–the temperature of a good refrigerator–the population of microbes usually doubles every thirty-five to forty hours. If there are too many microbes to start with, after several days of normal storage the numbers will be enormous. The investigators from Consumers Union found that seven samples tested had bacterial counts in excess of 130,000 per milliliter. One sample had almost 3 million and some had too many to count.

These organisms may well be harmless. They may not. The point is that some milks have a great number of microbes in them and you, the consumer, don't know how many you are buying.

If the findings of poor taste and bacterial contamination aren't enough to discourage the avid milk drinker, the investigators from Consumers Union found even more. Only four of twenty-five milk samples tested contained no detectable amounts of pesticide. The other twenty-one contained residues of chlorinated hydrocarbons, which are believed to be hazards to human health. There is increasing evidence to suggest that as they accumulate in the body they may produce mutations resulting in birth defects. These same hydrocarbons may also produce cancer.

Consumer Reports acknowledges that the level of pesticide contamination found in the milks was below the "action" limits established by the Food and Drug Administration. The FDA operates on the notion that a little bit of cancer-producing material won't hurt you. Many scientists, however, believe that no amount is safe. The Consumers Union expert milk consultant "considers the milk supply throughout the five-state Midwestern area covered in our tests to pose a potential hazard."

In their studies the Consumers Union investigators found no milks contaminated with antibiotics or aflatoxin. (Aflatoxin is a poisonous substance contained in moldy animal feed that can produce cancer in mammals. If a cow eats moldy feeds, aflatoxin will appear in the milk. Fortunately for milk drinkers this is an unusual contaminant.) Antibiotics, most commonly penicillin, are given to cows for the treatment of mastitis, an inflammation of the udders. Cows are not supposed to be milked for forty-eight hours after receiving penicillin. Often this precaution is not followed and then penicillin appears in the milk in small quantities.

People allergic to penicillin–an estimated 1 percent of the United States population–may develop symptoms of penicillin allergy after drinking milk contaminated with this antibiotic. The allergic reaction may take the form of hives, sneezing, asthma, or an unexplained rash.

Another naturally occurring substance in many cow milks is the hormone progesterone. This appears in the milk of pregnant cows. As pointed out by Dr. Jerome Fisher, "About 80 percent of cows that are giving milk are pregnant and are throwing off hormones continuously."

Progesterone breaks down into androgens, which have been implicated as a factor in the development of acne. Acne, as anyone who has reached the third decade of life can remember, is the scourge of adolescents. Adolescence also is a time when milk consumption may be enormous. Some teenagers pride themselves on drinking three or four quarts of milk a day. Dr. Fisher observed that his teenage acne patients drank much more milk than the rest of the general population. More importantly, he found that the acne improved as soon as the milk drinking stopped. Not all dermatologists agree with Dr. Fisher's hypothesis that hormones in milk are responsible for acne in adolescence, but many feel there is merit to the proposal that it may be at least one responsible factor in this poorly understood and potentially disfiguring disease.

Consumers Union gave whole cow milk a second chance and reported their findings in the June, 1982, issue of *Consumer's Report*. The article was entitled "Milk–Could it Taste Better?–Could it Cost Less? The answers to these questions, simply put, was "yes" and "yes."

The investigators found coliform bacteria in somewhat less than one-half of the samples tested. They state, "In no case can we say that the bacterial counts we found imply a public health hazard. Astronomic counts of benign bacteria can still be safe, while much lower counts of disease producers may pose a real danger. Still, bacterial counts are rough indicators of milk's sanitary qualities. High counts also usually mean rapid spoilage."

The survey revealed no "significant" residues of either chlorinated hydrocarbon pesticides or antibiotics. The writers of the article did not explain what was the meaning of the term "significant."

Consumers Union analyzed 40 samples of whole milk and found that 28 percent of the samples tested didn't contain enough fat to meet the standards of the state in which they were bought and about 30 percent fell short in terms of total solids, nonfat solids, or both. Their conclusion—"a good number of samples would shortchange milk drinkers both in flavor and nutritional value."

The investigation also revealed that the sodium content of the various milk categories tested to be about 25 to 40 milligrams higher than the figures published by the United States Department of Agriculture; bad news for people on low sodium diets.

The survey also identified great variation in milk out-dating policies. In some states, most notable the North-Central states, milk by the expiration date was judged to taste excellent or very good in only two out of every three samples tested. In these areas only 18 percent of the samples received high marks for taste when tested five days after the expiration date.

We now have come full circle. Not only is there very little evidence that cow milk is of nutritional benefit to humans, but it may not always taste good, may be contaminated with bacteria, and can contain substances that are actually hazardous to your health.

Does your milk taste different lately?

Chapter 8

"Beware of the Cow"

Diarrhea and cramps, gastrointestinal bleeding, iron-deficiency anemia, skin rashes, atherosclerosis, and acne. These are disorders that have been linked to the drinking of whole cow milk. So have recurrent ear infections and bronchitis. Can there be more? Yes. Leukemia, multiple sclerosis, rheumatoid arthritis, and simple dental decay have also been proposed as candidates.

Until now I have dealt with well-established facts. Now I would like to provide the reader with a number of very disturbing theories—disturbing, that is, only if you are still drinking milk.

A highly respected British medical journal, *The Lancet*, recently published an editorial review entitled "Beware of the Cow." The first sentence of this article read as follows: "Along with the evidence that beef-eating may be connected, in adults, with large-bowel cancer comes news of a possible fresh menace from cows, this time to the young."

The editorial went on to describe the report of an experiment in which unpasteurized cow milk was fed to baby chimpanzees—and two of six of these infant chimpanzees developed leukemia and died. Leukemia had never before been observed in chimpanzees. It must be noted that the milk given to these chimpanzees was special. It had come from cows known to be infected with a virus. This virus, called bovine C-type virus, is a natural infection of cows, and is believed to cause a form of leukemia in cattle.

This form of bovine leukemia was first recognized at the beginning of the twentieth century in Europe. It was quickly realized to be worldwide in its distribution, affecting all bovine races. It is known to be infectious among cattle and seems to be most capable of producing leukemia among those cows and bulls that appear to have a genetic predisposition to the disease. The virus had been transmitted to sheep but never before to a species so closely related to man.

In chimpanzee experiments six infants were fed milk from infected cows from the time of birth, while an additional six infants were fed milk from non-infected cows. Two of the chimps who received the infected milk died at thirty-four and thirty-five weeks of age after a six-week illness. They were found to have the bovine form of leukemia as well as an unusual type of infectious pneumonia.

Most infections that can be transmitted to chimpanzees can also be transmitted to human beings. At present there is no evidence that bovine C-type virus has ever been transmitted to humans. But the possibility remains and hence *The Lancet's* warning, "Beware of the Cow."

More on this disturbing prospect was raised by a report in *Science* by Doctors Farrar, Kenyon and Gupta, all from the University of Pennsylvania School of Veterinary Medicine. Milk, or living cells collected from the milk, of 24 dairy cattle, known to be naturally infected with bovine leukemia virus, was injected into lambs. The lambs were then examined for evidence of infection. Using this as a form of bioassay, infectious virus was demonstrated in the milk of 17 of the 24 cows tested. This infectivity is believed to be destroyed when milk is pasteurized. The authors nevertheless conclude with the following, "While earlier epidemiological surveys showed no association between human and bovine leukemia, the most recent survey, involving a large number of cases, showed a statistically significant increase in human acute lymphoid leukemia in areas with a high incidence of bovine leukemia and bovine leukemia virus infection. Clearly, the question of whether bovine leukemia virus poses a public health hazard deserves thorough investigation with the most sensitive virological and immunological techniques available...." Their words, not mine.

What about multiple sclerosis? Multiple sclerosis is a relentlessly progressive neurological disease which produces disturbances in speech, vision, and muscle function. Victims ultimately become invalids. Multiple sclerosis has a peculiar geographical distribution that has never been adequately explained. Within a large country such as the United States, multiple sclerosis is much more common in colder climates. Evidence from around the world suggests that multiple sclerosis rarely occurs near the equator. It has been proposed by many investigators that multiple sclerosis is caused by a virus and attacks individuals who have an alteration in their immunity.

Because of the unusual geographic distribution of this disease, two scientists from the University of Michigan, Drs. Bernard Agranoff and David Goldberg, began in 1974 to look for links between geography and other factors that might provide clues to how this disease is acquired.

These scientists studied the distribution of deaths of about 26,000 persons with multiple sclerosis in the United States. States like Alabama, Georgia, and Tennessee had only about half the number of cases that might otherwise have been predicted on the basis of population alone. Some striking relationships, both negative and positive, between multiple sclerosis and certain factors were observed. For example, no correlation was found between the incidence of multiple sclerosis and wealth, education, the number of physicians, hospitals, hospital beds, or nursing homes in an area. But the incidence of multiple sclerosis correlated most strikingly with a relatively low per-capita milk consumption.

Agranoff and Goldberg were excited. They next looked for similar relationships in other countries. They studied twenty-one other nations. Again they found that in these other twenty-one countries the only significant link was between multiple sclerosis and average milk consumption.

It is unclear, as yet, how milk consumption tends to increase the risk of developing multiple sclerosis. The investigators postulate that it might be a result of the fats in milk altering the nervous system of people who drink a lot of milk or possibly the presence of an unrecognized toxic substance or infectious agent. The investigators recognize that more work must be done to substantiate their theory. They close the account of their study with a phrase that bears a striking similarity to the advice given in the previously mentioned

Lancet editorial: "Cow's milk may be an unfortunate substitute for human milk in infancy or a risky food source thereafter, or both."

It may be more than coincidence that a group of investigators from the Baylor College of Medicine in Houston, Texas, also identified milk consumption as a factor in still another poorly understood neurological disease. This disease is amyotrophic lateral sclerosis—also popularly known as "Lou Gehrig disease" after the famous athlete who was a victim of this disorder. The neurologists analyzed many variables in twenty-five patients with this disease and compared the patients' histories with twenty-five healthy individuals of similar sex, age, racial background, economic status, and education. The factors that set apart the patients with amyotrophic lateral sclerosis from their normal counterparts was that the patients reported an increased incidence of exposure to lead and mercury, more participation in sports, and higher ingestion of cow milk. More food for thought.

Dr. J. Dan Baggett, the pediatrician from Montgomery, Alabama, who has so carefully observed the consequence of diet in his young patients, believes there is a link between the drinking of cow milk and the development of juvenile rheumatoid arthritis. He writes,

> *"In my experience, I have had several children with signs and symptoms of early rheumatoid arthritis, some of them having progressed with this to the point of alarming their parents and myself. Without exception, during the past eight years, I have had the good fortune to relieve them and watch their certain return to good health by simply eliminating all traces of milk from their diet. One child, now in my practice, after being diagnosed and treated as*

> *a definite rheumatoid arthritic by a renowned
> rheumatologist, has enjoyed dramatic
> improvement by having milk deleted from her
> diet."*

Many other pediatricians have had similar isolated
experiences. The pain and joint swelling of rheumatoid arthritis may be yet another manifestation of milk
allergy–an allergy that takes many subtle and puzzling forms.

Another bizarre and puzzling observation was reported by investigators in Tacoma, Washington. Alexander Schauss and co-workers found an apparent
relationship between heavy milk drinking and
anti-social behavior. When the diets of young crimi-
nals were contrasted with those of adolescents from a
similar background, it was found that the juvenile de-
linquents consumed almost ten times the amount of
milk that was drunk by the control group. The juvenile offenders ate less fruit, nuts and vegetables.
Schauss, who is continuing this investigation, was un-
certain if the consumption of large quantities of milk
produced some form of "protein intoxication" that resulted in crime or reflected an imbalanced diet that
were merely co-incidental. "Who knows what evil
lurks in the minds (or stomachs) of men?"

A real irony is that milk may actually lead to tooth
decay. Most mothers give cow milk to their infants in
an attempt to build strong teeth and strong bones. Dr.
Frances Castano, a dental researcher at the University of Pennsylvania, believes that under certain circumstances the drinking of milk may actually help
destroy the teeth. Many mothers get their baby to go
to sleep by providing him with a bottle at bedtime.
The baby contentedly sucks on the nipple and dozes
off. Then the trouble begins. After the baby has

stopped swallowing the milk, the milk begins to eat away at the teeth.

During sleep the secretion of saliva is markedly decreased. Milk in the mouth is neither digested nor washed away and instead remains on the teeth and turns sour. This soured milk serves as an excellent nutrient for the bacteria that inhabit the mouth. These same bacteria are responsible for the dental plaque formation that produces dental smooth-surface decay. According to Dr. Castano, the result of this bedtime practice is that decay can be so rapid that parents will report the teeth seem to be "melting away." This is particularly true when such feeding practices are continued after a baby is more than twelve months of age.

Dr. Castano strongly advocates breast feeding as a means of preventing this problem. If a bottle must be given at bedtime it should be filled with water.

Perhaps if we all drank more water, rather than whole cow milk, many of the diseases described in this chapter would also "melt away."

Chapter 9

"Milk Has Something for Everybody"

"Milk Drinkers Make Better Lovers"..."Everybody Needs Milk"..."Milk: Drink It for All It's Worth"..."There Is a New You Coming Every Day–Drink Milk"..."Milk– The Perfect Food."

You have probably seen one or more of these advertising slogans sponsored by the milk industry. But did you see the headline in an April, 1974, issue of the *New York Times* which announced "Federal Trade Commission Finds Milk Advertising Campaign Deceptive?" Most people who saw it probably didn't read it—and those who did read it probably didn't believe it.

In 1974 the Federal Trade Commission finally began to catch up with the dairy industry. Specifically, the FTC issued a "proposed complaint" against the California Milk Producers Advisory Board and

Cunningham and Walsh, its advertising agency. In the complaint they charged that the dairymen's campaign to stimulate milk sales constituted false, misleading, and deceptive advertising.

The dairy industry was shocked. After all, what had they done other than to proclaim that "Everybody Needs Milk?" The public has heard that line for years. This time the FTC wasn't buying the slogan. They couldn't. Too much scientific evidence had been accumulated which indicated that people didn't need milk and, in fact, that it could be harmful to your health. The complaint cited many of the facts I've reported in this book: the high incidence of lactase deficiency in the population; the frequency of cow milk allergy in children; the risks of heart disease from milk consumption.

The FTC complaint came in the midst of a massive campaign to stimulate lagging milk sales. The "California-Oregon-Washington Dairymen" had initiated a promotional blitz using radio, television, and newspaper ads. Promoting the slogan "Everybody Needs Milk" were such celebrities as Mark Spitz, Vida Blue, Ray Bolger, Abigail Van Buren, and Florence Henderson.

Abigail Van Buren suggested that drinking milk helped her avoid catching colds. Ray Bolger suggested that drinking milk was partially responsible for his long career as a dancer because it prevented him from developing arthritic joints.

How could these idols be wrong? We expect sage counsel when we ask a question of "Dear Abby." Vida Blue could not have won twenty games a season and Mark Spitz could not have collected all those Olympic medals if they didn't know the right things to eat.

It was an attractive campaign, but it was incorrect. The dairymen were fast on their feet. By the time the Federal Trade Commission had announced its intent to file a complaint, the advertising slogan had already been changed from "Everybody Needs Milk" to "Milk Has Something for Everybody." Who can argue with that?

Of course that "something" might be diarrhea, iron-deficiency anemia, or even a heart attack.

All this advertising eventually is reflected in the price you pay for milk. The farmer pays, and the consumer pays. Dairy farmers are, in fact, taxing themselves to raise revenues for these aggressive advertising campaigns. Last year New York state's dairy farmers voted to tax themselves up to $5 million a year to promote milk sales. These farmers own more than a million cows—cows that produce about ten and a half billion pounds of milk each year.

They were well aware that New Yorkers weren't drinking as much milk as they used to. Twenty-five years ago a resident of New York drank an average of one pint of milk per day; now a citizen of New York was drinking only slightly more than two-thirds of a pint per day. This change in drinking habits represents a decline of thirty quarts per person per year, or more than eleven million gallons a year.

The farmers were willing to tax themselves because the American Dairy Association provided them with information that was encouraging. A study by the association indicated that the investment of 15 cents per person for advertising in a milk marketing area will produce a return of $1.68 in new revenues. Remember the next time you hear a jingle praising the merits of milk—that's no "public service" announcement.

The action of the Federal Trade Commission in California was a monumental event for still another reason. Traditionally the federal government and the milk industry have worked together in promoting the sale of milk. A typical example of this cooperation is a pamphlet entitled, "Milk in Family Meals," published by the U.S. Department of Agriculture. This guide for homemakers starts off with the statement, "Milk is a basic food that everyone in the family needs every day." No wonder the milk industry was shocked by the complaint lodged by the Federal Trade Commission!

By the way, the pamphlet "Milk in Family Meals" was published by the U.S. Government Printing Office, an office supported by your tax dollars. The document superseded a publication, Home and Garden Bulletin 57, entitled "Getting Enough Milk," also written to encourage milk drinking by the American public.

The National Dairy Council serves as a watchdog designed to counter the claims of anyone foolish enough or un-American enough to question the virtues of milk. The National Dairy Council is governed by a sixty-member board of directors, made up of representatives of milk producers, milk processors, milk distributors, and manufacturers and jobbers of dairy supplies and equipment. Although their central office is located in Chicago, through subscription to news-clipping services they manage to survey every hamlet in the country for evidence of heresy.

Each time I have personally questioned the value of cow milk and the story reached the local press–be it in Baltimore, Philadelphia, Dallas, Syracuse, or Lancaster, Pennsylvania–the clipping rapidly reached the central office of the National Dairy Council in Chicago. As predictably as an echo from a cavern I would receive a letter from the council condemning my statements. Generally a letter from the Council would also appear in the newspaper carrying the story, criticizing it for printing the story and going to great lengths to defend the merits of milk.

It is difficult for an individual to fight an industry, especially one long protected by the government. Fortunately the scientific facts are slowly beginning to emerge. The milk industry continues to defend their product as perfect while at the same time it modifies it.

The frustrations of fighting the American belief in milk are well summarized by Dr. Ellen Mackenzie, who has been trained in pediatrics as well as psychiatry. In an article entitled "Psychologic Factors in Milk Anemia:" she writes:

> *"'Everybody needs milk,' carols a current commercial from television and billboards. Cow's milk, a liquid protein food well suited to a calf before its teeth erupt, has been so touted as "nature's most nearly perfect food" that even some doctors consider it an adequate substitute for a varied diet. The mystique of whole, homogenized, pasteurized, bottled milk (the most germ-laden, allergenic, and expensive of available formulas) is enormously powerful. Families will resume giving it despite their own experience or the doctor's warning of allergy, respiratory disease, or anemia. Mammon always intrudes: the director of a local television program was not allowed to mention milk anemia on his program because the dairy companies were big advertisers."*

Chapter 10

Milk and the Tension-Fatigue Syndrome

"You'll also see children whose parents bring them in for a checkup because a teacher may have complained, 'Johnny is so tired and sluggish, I wonder if he is getting enough rest.' And you'll see other children whose mothers say, 'Mike is so hyperactive and irritable; there are days when I simply can't stand him.' Such children may also experience trouble in learning and in getting along with siblings, schoolmates and teachers...."

William G. Crook
in *"Food Allergy-the Great Masquerader,"*
Pediatric Clinics of North America,
February, 1975

Most people, including physicians, believe that allergies to foods (as well as inhalants and drugs) produce only such classical symptoms as skin rashes, respiratory symptoms, or gastrointestinal disorders. There is a growing body of evidence, however, to suggest that certain allergies may manifest themselves primarily as changes in personality, emotions, or in one's general sense of well-being.

Dr. Crook, a pediatrician with over twenty years of experience in practice, has seen over four thousand children with complaints that can be attributed to food allergies. He believes that the foods that are the most common offenders are milk, corn, and cane sugar, and he is far from alone in this conviction.

What are the symptoms and what can be done to prove the relationship between food and the problem?

The child or adult with motor fatigue always seems to feel weak and tired. The child may interrupt his play in order to rest or may even have to put his head down on the desk at school because he is feeling so tired. Excessive drowsiness and torpor are typical. These children are particularly listless in the morning. They are difficult to awaken and appear never to have had a good night's sleep.

Anyone who has suffered from hay fever may appreciate this sensation. The English physician Charles Blackley first described the emotional component of this allergy in a series of experiments performed in 1873. He noted that the inhalation of pollen caused "a violent attack of sneezing" and "a copious discharge of thin serum" from his nose, and that in the course of several hours he developed a "sense of weariness over the whole body."

Obviously, not all children who suffer from chronic fatigue do so as a result of food allergy. Anemia, infections, or other chronic illnesses should be considered as possible causes before it is concluded that food allergy is responsible. But food allergy will prove to be more commonly responsible than these other serious diseases.

Tension is the other major manifestation of food allergy. These children will appear restless and in a constant state of activity. They fidget, grimace, twist, turn, jump, and just never seem to sit still. Many of these children are also excessively irritable and can never be pleased.

Although the "tension-fatigue" syndrome is the most common manifestation of food allergy, it is by no means the only one. Vague recurrent abdominal pains, repeated headaches, aching muscles and joints, and even bed-wetting have been observed as symptoms of food allergy.

Many children who suffer from these food allergies characteristically appear pale and have large circles under their eyes. They may have a nose that seems to be "stuffed" all the time.

Although I have emphasized the role played by food allergies in producing symptoms in children, adults appear equally prone to the problems produced by foods. Dr. H. L. Newbold, a psychiatrist, has identified many patients in his practice whose insomnia, anxiety, or depression has been produced by foods. The food most responsible for the symptoms in both adults and children is whole cow milk.

An example of the magnitude of this problem is provided by the experience of Dr. Crook. During an eight-month period, forty-five children were seen in his office with complaints of either hyperactivity or learning difficulties in school In forty-one of these forty-five children it could be demonstrated that the symptoms were produced by a food allergy. In these children the symptoms were partially or totally relieved when the offending food was removed from the diet.

Dr. Crook found that each child was allergic to an average of three foods. In this group of forty-one children, twenty-eight were sensitive to milk. Sensitivity to cane sugars was equally frequent; sensitivity to eggs, wheat, and corn were also common.

Food allergy should be suspected when symptoms of tension and fatigue are present, particularly in conjunction with pallor and a stuffed nose.

Dr. Crook recommends removal of the possible offending food for seven to twenty-one days. If food is responsible, the symptoms will dramatically improve during this brief interval. Reintroducing the food in the diet should produce a return of the original symptoms.

The first food to be removed is whole cow milk and all recipes and products that contain it.

Chapter 11

"What to Do Instead"

"A pair of substantial mammary glands has the advantage over the two hemispheres of the most learned professor's brain in the art of compounding a nutritious fluid for infants."

Oliver Wendell Holmes

This remark by Chief Justice Holmes is just as true today as it was at the turn of the century. But what about the woman who doesn't want to, or cannot, breast-feed her infant? What about the older child or the adult? What are they to drink if they don't drink cow milk? In this chapter I would like to discuss the substitutes for whole milk that are readily available to everyone.

The alternatives for infants presents no real problem. Although, as indicated previously, no commercial infant formula provides the protection against infection that is present in human breast milk, they all provide adequate nutrition for the baby during the first twelve months of life.

Similac, Enfamil, and SMA are the brand names of the three most popular infant formulas currently in use in the United States. All have been significantly modified from the cow milk from which they are derived. Each manufacturer has attempted to modify its product so that it resembles human milk as closely as possible in its composition of fat, protein, carbohydrate, and minerals. All three products have been demonstrated to provide adequate nutrition in infants.

All these commercial formulas are supplemented with vitamins and iron. All are capable of meeting an infant's needs during the first year of life. An infant who is not breast-fed should receive one of these formulas. Again: an infant should not be fed whole cow milk at any time during infancy.

The protein in these formulas is still derived from the protein of cow milk, even though it has been altered in processing. It is much less likely to produce the allergic symptoms and gastrointestinal irritation recognized to be hazards of whole cow milk. Some infants, nevertheless, will be allergic to the protein in these commercial formulas. For such infants, formulas derived from soy beans should be employed. These soybean formulas are also commercially available and have been shown to support good growth in babies. Some extremely allergic babies will even have symptoms while drinking soybean milks. These babies can be offered formulas which contain only the breakdown products of protein, amino acids. Such elemental formulas will support adequate nutrition in infants who do not tolerate other forms of feeding.

Most pediatric nutritionists believe that it is inadvisable to feed infants skim milk during the first year of life. Skim milk has had the fat of milk removed. Normally, during infancy, 35 to 55 percent of the calories an infant receives are in the form of fat. When skim milk is fed to infants very few calories are derived from fat. Instead, most of the calories come from protein and carbohydrate. Nutritionists are still concerned about the long-term consequences of removing fat from the diet so early in life.

In addition, an infant who is depending on skim milk as his primary source of nutrition is taking in larger quantities of minerals. This imbalance may also prove harmful. Dr. Samuel J. Fomon, universally regarded as an expert in the field of infant nutrition, recommends the following: "When attempts are made to control weight during infancy, it is recommended that modest rather than drastic reduction in calorie intake be employed. The diet should provide 7 to 16 percent of calories from protein and 35 to 55 percent of calories from fat. These dietary stipulations can be met with ease when human milk or whole cow milk (or infant formulas) serves as a major source of calories but are nearly impossible to meet when skim milk is fed."

Solid foods should gradually be reintroduced into the diet, starting at about five to six months of age. Fruits and cereals are usually fed first. Between six and nine months of age vegetables and meats may be offered. Eggs are best saved until last and should be added to the diet between nine months and one year of age. By the time an infant has reached one year most of his nutritional needs can be met by solid foods. Milk is no longer necessary. Juices, which can be begun early in life, provide extra fluid and extra calories in the form of carbohydrates.

After the age of one year the volume of commercial infant formula should be reduced so that by eighteen months of age the infant is no longer drinking milk of any kind.

What about the older members of our population? What are they drinking now? In 1975 the average American consumed the following:

Water	56.7 gallons
Soft drinks	39.6 gallons
Coffee	27.8 gallons
Beer	24.8 gallons
Milk	21.6 gallons
Tea	7.4 gallons
Juices	6.1 gallons
Distilled spirits	2.0 gallons
Wine	1.7 gallons

A quick review of these numbers indicates that the average American is drinking only about one gallon of water per week. Water consumption should certainly be encouraged. The drinking of fruit juices, which taste good and are also good for you, should also be increased.

If you are still not ready to give up milk or its close relatives, what is available?

The standard product, the cause of all the problems, is called grade A pasteurized milk. The U.S. Public Health Service has set standards for grade A pasteurized milk and milk products. To earn this grade, whole milk must contain not less than 3.25 percent milk fat and not less than 8.25 percent nonfat milk solids. These nonfat milk solids are the protein and carbohydrate. If milk is to be labeled grade A and shipped across state lines, it must meet these standards. Different standards are employed for labeling milks that are produced and sold within a state.

Grade A milk contains the fat that should be of concern to all adults. Grade A milk has the lactose that produces adverse symptoms for most of the world's population. Grade A milk also has the unmodified protein that is allergenic to many infants.

If you are an adult who can tolerate lactose, have no problems with allergic symptoms from milk proteins, and only wish to reduce your fat intake, then skim milk is the product for you. Skim or nonfat milk has less than 0.5 percent milk fat in it. The removal of the fat also removes the vitamin A. Some products are therefore fortified with vitamin A. Check the label to be sure.

Powdered milk is marketed as powdered whole milk or powdered skim milk. Both have had most of their water removed. The powdered skim milk has also had most of the fat removed before it is dried. Powdered milk of either variety is much less expensive than the fluid form from which it is derived. In general, powdered milk costs only one-third as much as whole milk. It possessed the same nutritional advantages of the liquid milk and produces the same problems as well.

Most people don't like the taste of the reconstituted powdered milk. This problem of taste can be largely overcome by mixing the milk with water and allowing it to stand in the refrigerator for twenty-four hours before drinking it. The cost savings of powdered milk may be worth the sacrifice in taste to some people.

Evaporated milk is prepared by removing about 60 percent of the water from fresh milk. Evaporated milk is made from either whole milk or skim milk. It is reconstituted by simply adding back the water. This milk is also cheaper than the fresh fluid form. The evaporation process tends to alter the protein of the milk slightly so that it may not be as allergenic to the infant with this problem. The sugar and fat are still present to cause difficulties.

Sweetened condensed milk is evaporated milk to which extra sugar has been added. This form of milk is generally used for baking and is not consumed in everyday drinking because of its excessive sweetness.

Filled milk is a milk or cream to which a fat other than butter fat has been added. A typical filled milk consists of skim milk or nonfat dry milk to which a (safer) vegetable fat has been added. Artificial color and flavor may be added as well. Filled milk looks, smells, and tastes like evaporated milk. It is cheaper and contains less cholesterol than whole milk.

Filled milk has had an interesting history in the United States. Its history reflects the power of the milk industry working in concert with the federal government. Fifty years ago Congress enacted legislation that prohibited the interstate transportation of filled milk. Charles Hauser, a dairy farmer from Litchfield, Illinois, fought the Filled Milk Act, as it came to be known. This manufacturer of filled milk spent hundreds of thousands of his own dollars in legal fees. He even went to jail for a weekend before being pardoned by President Franklin Roosevelt. Hauser was convinced that filled milk was a safe, wholesome product.

This "bastard" form of milk was a threat to the dairy industry. If people were allowed to tamper with whole milk the public would begin to ask questions about the "perfect nature" of the product. Congress, by passing legislation which banned interstate commerce in filled milk, placed men like Hauser and his Milnot Company at an economic disadvantage.

In 1973 the federal courts ruled that the Filled Milk Act was unconstitutional. The Food and Drug

Administration declared that filled milk is a safe, wholesome, and proper food. Scientists have urged for years that dairy products with milk fat removed are better for you. It took fifty years for Charles Hauser to be vindicated. The modification of milk now has both legal and scientific sanction.

Yogurt is another modified milk product that has begun to gain wide acceptance in this country. It has long been popular in the Middle East. Yogurt can be made from either skim milk or whole milk. It is better made from skim milk. Yogurt is made by combining skim milk with a bacterial culture and allowing the culture to ferment the milk. In the process of fermentation the lactose in the milk is broken down into its simple sugars, glucose and galactose. The bacteria do the job that the digestive enzymes of the gastrointestinal tract might otherwise do. The result is that lactose are reduced in yogurt and butter milk and many individuals with "lactose intolerance" can consume these without discomfort.

The removal of the fat also eliminates another of the disadvantages of whole milk. The culturing and incubation process is believed to modify the protein and reduce its chances of producing allergic symptoms. Yogurt, and not whole milk, may be closer to a "perfect food." Isn't that just what your grandmother told you?

Non-dairy imitation milks are also available. These products resemble milk but contain no complete milk ingredients. A typical imitation milk contains sodium caseinate (as the protein source), vegetable fat, corn syrup or dextrose, artificial color and flavor, and emulsifiers. Coffee lighteners or whiteners are a form of imitation milk. Sodium caseinate, although it originates from the cow, has been legally classified as a non-dairy ingredient because it has undergone changes and no longer simulates the calcium caseinate of whole milk from which it was derived. Sodium caseinate is soluble in water and forms a soft, easily digestible curd while calcium caseinate is soluble in water and forms a tough curd.

Robert E. Rich, Sr., is the founder of the Rich Products Corporation of Buffalo, New York, the initial developer of imitation cream. Rich hopes that "Someday you may have to go to the zoo to see a cow." Rich feels that the so-called imitations are not really imitations but are, in fact, functionally superior to the real thing. They are made from soybeans or other beans or other oils and various chemicals. They are sold frozen, and they won't curdle, separate, or sour even weeks after being thawed. They are cheaper to begin with and they save money on spoilage and refrigeration.

Rich developed his product in 1945. He was in the dairy business then but already had become disenchanted with the cow as a means of making a livelihood. "We already knew the cow was a pretty poor economic creature. The supply is unreliable, and the quality varies. Besides, milk is susceptible to bacteria and it's 87 percent water—very inefficient," he said in an interview with *Forbes* magazine.

The dairy industry is slowly acknowledging that its product is not perfect. They have introduced skim milk to quiet the alarms of nutritionists about the danger of too much fat in the American diet. They are experimenting with milks in which the lactose has been altered so that it won't produce digestive difficulties for so many people.

In addition, research workers at the Massachusetts Institute of Technology are performing experiments on mice in an effort to solve the problem of lactose intolerance. Employing another approach, they are adding the enzyme lactase to milk. The enzyme is obtained from yeast that is designed to replace the enzyme that is missing from the human intestinal tract. It appears to work in mice, but hasn't yet been tried in humans as of this writing. Thought has also been given to altering the protein to reduce its allergic threat. In the not too distant future milk may be so transformed that you won't be able to recognize it.

The future may, in fact, be here right now. A product derived from milk, preserving the good but removing the bad, has been developed. Much of the credit for this whey-predominant milk must go to Roy Brog, the son of a Wyoming cheese-maker. For over twenty years Brog, now living in Utah, experimented with whey to produce a drink that had just the right taste and essentially no milk fat, 40 percent less lactose, and was potentially less allergenic than whole cow milk. During the last decade this type of whey-predominant milk has become commercially available. Why whey?

All mammalian milks have 2 major classes of protein—the whey and curd factions. Do you remember Little Miss Muffet who sat on her tuffet eating "her curds and whey?" The curd faction of milk is comprised of a variety of milk proteins termed caseins while the whey proteins include lactoferrin, alpha-lactoglobulin, beta-lactoglobulin, albumin, lysozyme, and immunoglobulins. Enzymatic or acid treatment of milk removes the curd. When casein is removed from skim milk the remaining portion is whey or "milk serum." Some states have erroneously classified it as a filled milk; however, filled milk by definition is cow milk with the animal fat replaced by a vegetable fat.

Human milk protein is approximately 80 percent whey and 20 percent curd or casein. Cow milk protein is almost precisely the opposite with slightly more than 80 percent of its protein being comprised of casein. The chemical composition of the whey and curd proteins of cow milk and human milk, however, are not identical. Whey proteins are believed to be nutritionally superior proteins. Infant formula manufacturers are now producing whey-predominate milks in recognition of this fact. It is one more step in their attempt to simulate human milk as much as possible. It was only logical that a whey-predominate milk would be made available for adult consumption as well.

Although whey predominate milks may vary in their other components, they, in general, have much less fat and less lactose than whole cow milk. Not only are these milks low in fat, but, unlike so-called two percent low fat milk, they also have less of the undesirable saturated fats per serving.

Because the whey predominate milks are manufactured, they may also be supplemented or fortified with minerals and vitamins that are not normally present in adequate quantities in natural whole cow milk. Because sweet whey milks deal with the nutritional problems that are a major source of concern of whole cow milk, such as too much fat, lactose intolerance, and protein intolerance, they present a threat to the leaders of the dairy industry. If milk is "a natural" how can you improve on "the perfect food?" Any improvement on whole cow milk is a tacit acknowledgment that it is not perfect.

What is the future for whole cow milk? Without the benefit of a crystal ball I can only guess. The trend, however, is obvious. Infants in the United States are now fed either human milk or a proprietary formula that simulates human milk in its composition. In 1971 approximately 68 percent of infants five to six months of age were drinking either whole cow milk or evaporated cow milk. In 1981, a short ten years later, the number of infants drinking whole milk at five to six months of age has fallen to only 17 percent. In another ten years it will be hard to find any infant exposed to the hazards of whole milk in the early months of life.

The picture is changing for the older child and the adult as well. The dairy industry is championing the cause for skim milk, low-fat milk, and low-lactose milks. They are in full retreat from their "perfect food" as wave upon wave of new scientific facts call into question the safety of whole cow milk.

In the future, whey-predominate milks will be the sole source of feeding for the infant who does not have the good fortune to be fed human milk. Whey-predominate formulas will be specially prepared to meet the unique nutritional requirements of infants. In a similar fashion, whey-predominate, low-fat, low-lactose milks will be widely used to feed adults. These filled milks will also be specially prepared and fortified to meet the nutritional requirements of older children and adults.

Cow milk has no valid claim as the perfect food. As nutrition, it produces allergies in infants, diarrhea and cramps in the older child and adult, and may be a factor in the development of heart attacks and strokes.

Perhaps when the public is educated as to the hazards of milk only calves will be left to drink the real thing. Only calves should drink the real thing.

Research Appendix

ANNALS OF INTERNAL MEDICINE[*]

Beer AE, Billingham RE "Immunologic benefits and hazards of milk in maternal-perinatal relationship." *Ann Intern Med* (1975 Dec) 83(6):865-71

Aside from nutritional significance, milk affords infant mammals immunologic benefits. However, it is not without immunologically based hazards. These stem from its antigenicity and the fact that in certain species that receive their maternal immunologic endowment postpartum, hemolytic disease of the newborn may be mediated by colostral antibodies.

---

[*] DATA SOURCES: The pertinent articles were identified using the Paper*Chase* database of Beth Israel Hospital, 350 Longwood avenue, Boston, MA 02115 Phone: 800/722-2075
MEDLINE, is indexed and abstracted by the National Institutes of Health, U.S. National Library of Medicine, Bethesda, MD 20894 Phone: 800/272-4787.

Awareness that viable leukocytes are ingredients of colostrum and milk has stimulated interest in the significance of these cells. Skin grafting tests on foster-nursed rats and mice have given circumstantial evidence that, in these species, leukocytes may be transmitted naturally from the mother's blood stream to the suckling's blood stream through the milk, and that these cells may be beneficial (adoptive immunization) or, in some genetic contexts, harmful (initiating graft-versus-host disease). In man, too, studies on necrotizing enteritis and other disease provide increasing support for the thesis that leukocytes in milk fulfill a protective function, possibly as a consequence of their "natural" transplantation.

ARCHIVES OF DISEASE IN CHILDHOOD

Burr ML "Does infant feeding affect the risk of allergy?" *Arch Dis Child* (1983 Jul) 58(7):561-5

For nearly 50 years the hypothesis has been debated that withholding cows' milk from babies reduces the risk of allergic disease. Numerous studies have been conducted of varying design, size, and quality, and with conflicting results. Evidence tends to favour the hypothesis, but the only firm conclusion that can be drawn is that random controlled trials with blind assessment are needed to settle the issue.

Minford AM, MacDonald A, Littlewood JM "Food intolerance and food allergy in children: a review of 68 cases." *Arch Dis Child* (1982 Oct) 57(10):742-7

The clinical and laboratory features of 68 children with food intolerance or food allergy are reviewed. Young children were affected the most with 79% first experiencing symptoms before age 1 year. Forty-eight

(70%) children presented with gastrointestinal symptoms (vomiting, diarrhoea, colic, abdominal pain, failure to thrive), 16 (24%) children with skin manifestations (eczema, urticaria, angioneurotic oedema, other rashes), and 4 (6%) children with wheeze. Twenty-one children had failed to thrive before diagnosis. A single food (most commonly cows' milk) was concerned in 28 (41%) cases. Forty (59%) children had multiple food intolerance or allergy; eggs, cows' milk, and wheat were the most common. Diagnosis was based on observing the effect of food withdrawal and of subsequent rechallenge. In many children food withdrawal will mean the use of an elimination diet which requires careful supervision by a dietician. Laboratory investigations were often unhelpful in suggesting or confirming the diagnosis.

CANCER RESEARCH

Correa P "EPIDEMIOLOGICAL CORRELATIONS BETWEEN DIET AND CANCER FREQUENCY" *Cancer Res* (1981) 41(9,part2):3685-3689

The literature concerning international correlations between dietary items and cancer frequency is reviewed. An updated correlation of the most recent data on cancer mortality and food consumption is made. Strong and consistent correlations are reported between death rates of cancers of the colon and breast and the per capita consumption of total fat and of nutrients derived from animal sources, especially beef, pork, eggs, and milk. Similar but less consistent correlations have been reported with cancers of the prostate, ovary, and endometrium. In addition, correlations between precursor lesions of coronary heart disease and colon cancer in New Orleans autopsy populations are reported. Some studies suggest that milk intake correlates better with atherosclerotic disease while beef intake correlates better with colon cancer. Negative correlations of colon cancer rates and vegetable consumption are reported. Colon cancer rates also show negative correlations with stool wt, irrespective of the type of vegetable responsible for the increased bulk. Epidemiological data are consistent with the hypothesis that excessive beef and low vegetable consumption are causally related to colon cancer. These food items probably do not have a direct carcinogenic role but rather provide a microenvironment favorable to the actions of carcinogens. (Author abstract) (47 Refs)

Institutional address: Louisiana State Univ. Medical Center
New Orleans LA 70112

CLINICAL PEDIATRICS

Wilson NW, Self TW, Hamburger RN "Severe cow's milk induced colitis in an exclusively breast-fed neonate. Case report and clinical review of cow's milk allergy." *Clin Pediatr* (Phila) (1990 Feb) 29(2):77-80

Cow's milk induced eosinophilic colitis presenting in the first week of life has been reported, but is very rare. The authors describe a 4- day-old female infant who presented with profuse rectal bleeding resulting in a hematocrit fall from 38% to 30% within 8 hr after hospital admission. Sigmoidoscopy revealed colonic mucosa that was red, edematous, and friable, with punctate hemorrhages. Rectal biopsy showed marked eosinophilic infiltration with multifocal hemorrhage. Further history indicated that while the infant had been exclusively breast-fed since birth, the nursing mother had been drinking 4-5 glasses of cow's milk per day since delivery. Prick puncture skin testing of the infant was positive for cow's milk protein. A serum radioallergosorbent test (RAST) for cow's milk protein was positive. The infant's serum IgE was 1.5 IU/ml. Rectal bleeding resolved when the patient was given a casein hydrolysate formula (Nutramigen, Mead Johnson Nutrition, Evansville, IN), and endoscopy one week later showed improvement, with only scattered areas of erythema, and no friability. We conclude that since the infant was exclusively breast- fed, the milk protein must have passed into the breast milk antigenically intact. Prenatal sensitization probably occurred. Cow's milk induced allergic colitis should be considered in the differential diagnosis of colitis in breast-fed neonates.

Institutional address: Department of Pediatrics
University of California
San Diego, La Jolla 92093.

JOURNAL OF FAMILY PRACTICE

Deamer WC, Gerrard JW, Speer F "Cow's milk allergy: a critical review." *J Fam Pract* (1979 Aug) 9(2):223-32

Foods which are ingested frequently, and cow's milk in particular, are a common cause of delayed-in-onset allergy. Difficulty in diagnosing milk allergy is encountered because: (1) skin tests are unreliable; (2) the symptoms of milk allergy are frequently delayed in appearing, thereby obscuring their connection with the previously ingested food; (3) when such symptoms do appear, they often fail to suggest allergy as etiologic; and (4) the offending antigen may be present in a milk product not obviously associated with milk per se such as sherbet or cheese. Contrary to common belief, most milk (and other food) allergy is not reagin (IgE) mediated. Milk allergy is not confined to infancy, but is frequently seen in children and adults, often persisting as an allergy which had supposedly been "outgrown." Since milk allergy is often a familial disorder, its presence in a patient can assist the physician in possibly discovering it in other members of the family. A two or three-week trial elimination of milk, in conjunction with written dietary instructions for the patient, is presently the only reliable diagnostic procedure.

JOURNAL OF PEDIATRICS

Brown KH "Dietary management of acute childhood diarrhea: optimal timing of feeding and appropriate use of milks and mixed diets." *J Pediatr* (1991 Apr) 118(4 (Pt 2)):S92-8

Several recent clinical trials have examined the optimal timing of feeding and the appropriate foods for use in the dietary management of acute childhood diarrhea. Important methodologic issues relevant to these trials, such as the composition and masking of study diets, measurement of outcome variables, and assessment of nutritional status, are discussed. Available data suggest that feeding should be continued during diarrhea, although a small subgroup of patients receiving nonhuman milk exclusively may have an excess rate of complications. These children should be closely supervised or provided with alternative diets. By contrast, children receiving human milk, nonmilk formulas, and mixed diets are generally able to tolerate these foods and to benefit nutritionally from continued feeding.

Institutional address: Department of Nutrition
University of California Davis 95616.

Kleinman RE "Cow milk allergy in infancy and hypoallergenic formulas." *J Pediatr* (1992 Nov) 121(5 Pt 2):S116-21

Substitute feedings have been used to treat infants with cow milk protein allergy for most of this century. For the past 50 years, several infant formulas based on animal proteins, both intact and chemically modified, or on vegetable protein have been labeled "hypoallergenic." Because of the risk of anaphylaxis and other serious adverse reactions, formulas that are claimed to be hypoallergenic should be subjected to rigorous preclinical and clinical testing. At a minimum, such formulas should not provoke any allergic signs or symptoms in 90% of infants with documented cow milk protein allergy when tested in double-blind, placebo-controlled trials. A standardized definition of "hypoallergenic" will allow clinicians and parents to understand the true risks to a cow milk- allergic infant fed such hypoallergenic formulas.

Institutional address: Combined Program in Pediatric
Gastroenterology and Nutrition
Harvard Medical School
Massachusetts General Hospital
Boston 02114.

PEDIATRICS

Oski FA "Is bovine milk a health hazard?" *Pediatrics* (1985 Jan) 75(1 Pt 2):182-6

Whole bovine milk should not be fed to infants during the first year of life because of its association with occult gastrointestinal bleeding, iron deficiency anemia, and cow's milk allergy. The consumption of whole milk after the first year of life should be discouraged because of its potential role in a variety of disorders including atherosclerosis, recurrent abdominal pain of childhood, cataracts, milk-borne infections, and juvenile delinquency.

Foucard T "Development of food allergies with special reference to cow's milk allergy." *Pediatrics* (1985 Jan) 75(1 Pt 2):177-81

Using strict criteria, the incidence of cow's milk sensitivity is probably 1% to 2% during the first 2 years of life. Although there is a wide spectrum of sensitivity symptoms caused by cow's milk, two major groups of infants are discernible. One group consists of infants who react to small amounts of cow's milk within a few minutes up to one hour, usually with gastrointestinal symptoms or urticaria. These infants are often atopic and have positive findings on skin prick tests and radioallergosorbent test (RAST) reactions to cow's milk allergens. The other group consists of children whose reaction to cow's milk occurs one hour or longer after intake of cow's milk or cow's milk-based formula. These reactions are usually not immunoglobulin (Ig)E-mediated and different immune and nonimmune mechanisms probably cause the symptoms. The risk of developing cow's milk sensitivity seems to be influenced by the atopic constitution of the infant and the age at which cow's milk is introduced. Early exposure to cow's milk increases the risk, not only of adverse reactions to this milk but also of developing allergies to other foods. It is suggested that early introduction of cow's milk may enhance the risk of future respiratory allergies. Allergists are still not in agreement as to whether the weaning process should be rapid or should consist of a gradual change from breast milk to cow's milk in order to minimize the risk of cow's milk allergy.

ACTA PAEDIATRICA. SUPPLEMENT

Lembcke JL, Brown KH "Effect of milk-containing diets on the severity and duration of childhood diarrhea." *Acta Paediatr Suppl* (1992 Sep) 381:87-92

Individual components of milk from humans and other mammalian species may influence the severity, duration, and nutritional outcome of childhood diarrhea in different ways. Nonetheless, empirical data from clinical trials can be used to assess children's responses to specific milk-containing diets. Factors modifying the response to milk include its source, amount, frequency of feeding, type of processing, and accompanying foods, as well as the type and severity of enteric infection and specific characteristics of the host. Whereas breast-fed infants have less severe diarrhea when breast milk is continued rather than interrupted, infants and children fed with non-human milks tend to have more severe illness than those receiving milk-free or lactose-limited formulas or milk-cereal mixtures. Fermentation of milk may reduce the severity of lactose malabsorption, but additional information regarding the efficacy of yogurt in acute, childhood diarrhea is still needed.

Don't Drink Your Milk!

Institutional address: Department of Nutrition
University of California Davis 95616-8669.

ANALES ESPANOLES DE PEDIATRIA

Escribano Subias J, Sanz Manrique N, Villa Elizaga I, Tormo Carnice R "[Relationship between primary lactose malabsorption and consumption of dairy products] Influencia de la hipolactasia primaria sobre el consumo de productos lacteos." *An Esp Pediatr* (1993 Feb) 38(2):107-12 (Published in Spanish)

This study was designed to determine the influence of lactose malabsorption on the consumption of dairy products. We studied 157 children and 43 adults. The Breath-hydrogen test was used to define their level of lactose digestion. The prevalence of lactose maldigesters was 12%. We found a large relationship between the consumption of milk and milk products and age. Malabsorbers consumed more fermented dairy products (ripened cheese and yogurt) than did absorbers (p 0.05). Subjects with normal lactose absorption consumed more milk, butter, cream cheese and global lactose than the maldigesters (p 0.05). Lactose intolerance, familiar consumption and geographic origins had little influence on an individual's consumption habits.

Institutional address: Servicio de Pediatria Hospital
Sant Joan de Reus Pamplona.

Lafuente Mesanza P, Ojembarrena Martinez E, Sasieta Altuna M, Pinan Frances MA, Urreta Dolora MJ, Lombardero Jimenez JL "[Anemia and depletion of iron reserves in healthy 12-month-old infants] Anemia y depleccion de depositos de hierro en lactantes sanos de 12 meses de edad." *An Esp Pediatr* (1992 Jul) 37(1):24-8 (Published in Spanish)

A prospective study was made which included 287 infants, 12 months of age and patients of two Vizcaya

Health Centers, in order to determine the prevalence of anemia and/or depletion of iron stores. The study design included somatometry and a review of the clinical records, dietary habits and the socio-economic status of the family. Laboratory tests included: hematocrit, hemoglobin, mean corpuscular volume, number of erythrocytes, serum iron, transferrin, iron saturation percentage and serum ferritin. Anemia was present in 9.3% of these children and 6.9% had iron-deficiency anemia. Depletion of iron stores was found in 12.4%. Prematurity, socio-economic status, infants fed low-iron milk, early introduction of cow's milk and the weight at 12 months were all variables that correlated significantly with the anemic or iron deficient states. However, the number of infections during the first year of life did not show a significant correlation. A question about the necessity of routine screening is raised and recommendation is made for iron supplementation in the infants in the high risk group.

Institutional address: Centro de Salud de Erandio
                    Desanexion Vizcaya.

ANNALS OF MEDICINE

Virtanen SM, Aro A "Dietary factors in the aetiology of diabetes."
Ann Med (1994 Dec) 26(6):469-78

Quite different nutrition-related environmental factors influence the development of type 1 insulin-dependent diabetes (IDDM) and type 2 non-insulin-dependent diabetes (NIDDM). IDDM is characterized by progressive beta-cell destruction which leads to complete insulin deficiency; at the time of diagnosis 80-90% of beta cells have been destroyed. In children there is epidemiological evidence that high intake of nitrites and N-nitroso compounds, early introduction of cow's milk to the diet and short duration or absence of breastfeeding increase the risk of IDDM. Studies in experimental animals suggest that cow's milk and soy proteins may be diabetogenic. There is current interest in the effects of free radical scavengers, particularly niacin and natural and synthetic antioxidants on the incidence of IDDM. These findings from ecological, animal, and human case-control studies remain to be evaluated in prospective cohort studies covering infancy and childhood and finally in human intervention trials. NIDDM is characterized by insulin resistance which is complicated by impaired insulin secretion at the time of appearance of hyperglycaemia and clinical diabetes. Its preclinical development is insidious and poorly defined, and there is little direct evidence that the same factors which influence metabolic control in clinical diabetes also affect the preclinical development of the disorder. Obesity, particularly of the abdominal type, is common in people who develop NIDDM, and weight control by appropriate diet and physical activity is probably the most important measure for preventing NIDDM. High (saturated) fat intake seems to be associated with insulin resistance, obesity and increased risk of NIDDM, and diets high in carbohydrate seem to protect from glucose intolerance and diabetes, mainly owing to their high fibre content.

Institutional address: Department of Applied Chemistry
and Microbiology University
of Helsinki Finland.

CRC CRITICAL REVIEWS IN FOOD SCIENCE AND NUTRITION

Lee VA, Lorenz K "The nutritional and physiological impact of milk in human nutrition." *CRC Crit Rev Food Sci Nutr* (1978) 11(1):41-116

The nutritional value of milk as an important source of energy, high- quality protein, calcium, and riboflavin has been recognized for many years. Currently, the widespread use and promotion of milk in the U.S. as well as developing countries has been questioned. This review examines the nutrient composition of dairy products, factors that account for variability in composition of milk, milk processing, preservation, quality control, and contaminants (such as minerals, radionuclides antibiotics, microorganisms and their metabolites, herbicides, and insecticides) in milk. Consumption patterns for milk and evidence for its nutritional value, especially in children, are presented. Milk consumption has been related to disease or conditions such as atherosclerosis, milk allergy, lactose intolerance, anemia, dental problems, and others. Recent recommendations for dietary changes for individuals in the U.S. and other developed countries could affect the use of milk. In addition, the use of feeding programs in the U.S. and developing countries which are based primarily on milk has been criticized. The preparation of new types of milk designed to offset certain difficulties encountered with cow's milk are now being evaluated in humans.

Don't Drink Your Milk!

CRITICAL REVIEWS IN FOOD SCIENCE AND NUTRITION

Jackson LS, Lee K "The effect of dairy products on iron availability." *Crit Rev Food Sci Nutr* (1992) 31(4):259-70

Many researchers report substantial reductions in iron availability when dairy products are consumed with solutions of iron. Yet other studies indicate that dairy products have little effect on iron availability when added to complex meals. The conflicting data may be due to differences in the technique used to measure availability, species of animal used, form of iron in the diet, and meal composition. Human studies show superior bioavailability of iron in human milk when compared with cow's milk. Definitive causes for the differences between human and cow's milk have not been identified. Human milk contains lower amounts of casein, phosphate, and calcium, components thought to inhibit iron absorption. More work is needed to identify the factors that influence iron-dairy interactions. The nutritional benefits provided by dairy products outweigh the slight inhibitory effect they may have on iron availability.

Institutional address: National Center for Food
Safety and Technology
Summit-Argo IL 60501.

DIABETES CARE

Gerstein HC "Cow's milk exposure and type I diabetes mellitus. A critical overview of the clinical literature." *Diabetes Care* (1994 Jan) 17(1):13-9

OBJECTIVE—To critically review and summarize the clinical evidence relating a short duration of breast-feeding or early cow's milk exposure to insulin-dependent (type I) diabetes. RESEARCH DESIGN AND METHODS—All relevant citations retrieved through comprehensive searching of the medical literature were critically reviewed and analyzed. Those case-control studies that minimized the possibility of bias were meta-analyzed to determine overall odds ratios (ORs) and 95% confidence intervals (CIs). RESULTS—Ecological and time-series studies consistently showed a relationship between type I diabetes and either cow's milk exposure or diminished breast-feeding. In the case-control studies, patients with type I diabetes were more likely to have been breast-fed for 3 months (overall OR 1.43; 95% CI 1.15-1.77) and to have been exposed to cow's milk before 4 months (overall OR 1.63; 95% CI 1.22-2.17). Slightly lower ORs were obtained when all of the case-control studies were meta-analyzed in a sensitivity analysis. CONCLUSIONS—Early cow's milk exposure may be an important determinant of subsequent type I diabetes and may increase the risk approximately 1.5 times.

Institutional address: Department of Medicine McMaster
University Hamilton Ontario Canada.

JOURNAL OF THE AMERICAN COLLEGE OF NUTRITION

Couet C, Jan P, Debry G "Lactose and cataract in humans: a review." *J Am Coll Nutr* (1991 Feb) 10(1):79-86

In this review, the relationship between lactose and human cataract is examined from the presently available biochemical, metabolic, and epidemiological data. The exceptional cases of homozygous enzyme deficiency being excluded, fragmentary data give reason to believe that a risk of cataract secondary to lactose and galactose ingestion is present in certain subpopulations. In these population groups, the size of which is unknown, the lens could be exposed to intermittent episodes of hypergalactosemia due to the presence of a partial enzyme deficiency in the galactose metabolic pathway, and/or the persistence of a high adult jejunal lactase activity, and/or to a large and repeated consumption of either whole lactose or easily absorbed lactose (hydrolyzed forms and nonpasteurized yogurt).

Institutional address: Clinique Medicale A Hopital
                              Bretonneau Tours France.

JOURNAL OF DAIRY SCIENCE

Deeth HC "Homogenized milk and atherosclerotic disease: a review." *J Dairy Sci* (1983 Jul) 66(7):1419-35

The theory that consumption of homogenized milk containing active xanthine oxidase is a causative factor in development of atherosclerosis is reviewed. Biologically available xanthine oxidase in consumed milk products may be absorbed in the small intestine and enter the blood stream. However, there appears to be no unequivocal evidence that the absorbed enzyme has any pathological effects that may contribute to development of atherosclerotic heart disease.

Garza C "Appropriateness of milk use in international supplementary feeding programs." *J Dairy Sci* (1979 Oct) 62(10):1673-84

Recognition of lactose intolerance, debate over the limitedness of dietary energy and protein in specific settings, and the appreciation for the uniqueness and appropriateness of human milk during the 1st yr of life have prompted reexamination of the use of milk in international feeding programs. Substantial proportions of preschool and school-age children from expected populations are lactose intolerant. However, studies in this county indicate that lactose intolerant preschool and early school-age children can tolerate amounts of milk usually consumed. Older individuals with symptomatic responses to milk also will often have similarly mild symptomatic responses to hydrolyzed lactose milk. Appropriately controlled studies in developing countries are planned or are underway to assess milk tolerance. In feeding programs designed to provide a protein supplement, milk continues to be a very attractive option. The question of how much milk protein must be given and how often it should be provided to make a significant impact on a population's well-being depends on an evaluation of the data base describing protein intakes and needs for specific populations. These types of data for most populations are inadequate.

JOURNAL OF DIARRHOEAL DISEASES RESEARCH

Brown KH, Lake A "Appropriate use of human and non-human milk for the dietary management of children with diarrhoea." *J Diarrhoeal Dis Res* (1991 Sep) 9(3):168-85

The nutritional benefit of milk consumption during diarrhoea must be balanced against its potential to produce increased severity or duration of illness. Continued breastfeeding during diarrhoea results in decreased stool output and is generally recommended. However, continued feeding of non-human milk may cause increased faecal excretion, prolonged diarrhoeal duration, and a greater number of treatment failures among young patients with relatively severe diarrhoea. Although most children can safely continue receiving milk during acute diarrhoea, the possibility of serious complications dictates that they be carefully observed. Acceptable alternatives to exclusive non-human milk feeding during diarrhoea include milk-free formulas, milk-cereal mixtures, and possibly fermented milks. This paper reviews the results of published clinical trials of milk feeding and discusses their implications for the appropriate dietary management of childhood diarrhoea.

Institutional address: Department of Nutrition
University of California Davis 95616.

KLINISCHE PADIATRIE

Harms HK "[Cow's milk protein sensitive enteropathy] Die kuhmilcheiweissabhangige Darmkrankheit des jungen Sauglings, eine Form der Kuhmilchproteinintoleranz." *Klin Padiatr* (1982 Nov-Dec) 194(6):375-80 (Published in German)

Cow's milk protein sensitive enteropathy (CMPSE) is characterized by the following items: 1. The great majority of affected infants have not been breast fed or only for a few days. Additional risks are immaturity, preceding enteritis, trisomy 21, and abdominal operation in the newborn. 2. Half of the patients become ill during the first two weeks after starting cow's milk formula. The main symptoms are watery, mucus containing diarrhea, vomiting, abdominal distension, pallor and rapid weight loss. 3. In CMPSE the small intestinal mucosa shows varying degrees of inflammation and villous atrophy. Bloody stools refer to large bowel affection. 4. CMPSE is always transitory and usually persists for less than one year. Inadequate treatment leads to "severe protracted diarrhea" or "intractable diarrhea" syndrome. Soya-based formula should not be the diet of first choice, since secondary intolerance to soya proteins will frequently develop. Exclusive breast feeding during the first months of life is the best prophylaxis of CMPSE.

MEDICAL HYPOTHESES

Ramabadran K, Bansinath M "Opioid peptides from milk as a possible cause of sudden infant death syndrome." *Med Hypotheses* (1988 Nov) 27(3):181-7

Milk from breast or baby formula is the exclusive source of nutrition for newborn infants. Short chain opioid peptides such as beta- casomorphins have been isolated from breast milk as well as baby formula. These biologically active peptides are absorbed from the gastrointestinal tract. In infants predisposed to respiratory apnea because of abnormal autonomic nervous system development and respiratory control mechanisms, opioid peptides derived from milk might be one of the etiological factors for sudden infant death syndrome and near miss sudden infant death syndrome.

Institutional address: Department of Anesthesiology
New York University Medical Center
NY 10016.

Rank P "Milk and arteriosclerosis." *Med Hypotheses* (1986 Jul) 20(3):317-38

Milk consumption is related to arteriosclerosis. Recent landmark studies confirm a previously suspected close correlation between milk intake and arteriosclerotic heart disease. Support is therefore provided for a recently proposed novel hypothesis that arteriosclerosis is a chronic infectious disease caused by blue-green bacteria and that milk is a carrier vehicle for these contaminant organisms. A revisionist view of diet and milk in the causation of arteriosclerosis is developed. Previous hypotheses relating milk consumption to arteriosclerosis and advances in pasteurization techniques are discussed and integrated with this infection theory.

Strand FT "Primary prevention of insulin-dependent diabetes mellitus: simple approaches using thermal modification of milk." *Med Hypotheses* (1994 Feb) 42(2):110-4

Evidence is presented that new cases of primary insulin dependent diabetes mellitus (IDDM) will cease to occur when milk-processing temperatures are increased from current levels (72 degrees C) to at least 85 degrees C. This temperature is sufficient to denature bovine serum albumin (BSA), the environmental trigger molecule for IDDM. Morbidity and mortality from atherosclerotic vascular disease (ASVD) and a number of autoimmune diseases may also be reduced by such increases in milk-processing temperatures. BSA-free milk products commercially available now include those canned (100 degrees C), ultrapasteurized (138 degrees C), and ultrahigh-temperature (UHT) processed (149 degrees C). At less than 6400 feet elevation, BSA can be denatured by simply bringing milk to a boil (85 degrees C). Until such time as all milk is routinely heat-treated to denature BSA, the safest course to maintain good nutrition and prevent IDDM and other BSA-triggered diseases is selection of milk products processed at temperatures above 85 degrees C.

Research Appendix

MONATSSCHRIFT FUR KINDERHEILKUNDE

Stern M "[Cow's milk protein intolerance: clinical and pathogenic aspects (author's transl)] Kuhmilchproteinintoleranz—Klinik und Pathogenese." *Monatsschr Kinderheilkd* (1981 Jan) 129(1):18-26 (Published in German)

Cow's milk protein intolerance is a transient food intolerance of early infancy. Ingestion of cow's milk protein causes an enteropathy of variable degree. Clinical manifestations are primarily gastrointestinal, although dermal and respiratory symptoms add to the clinical syndrome. Three types are found: an acute anaphylactic reaction, a chronic mild form, and a chronic severe form which is of utmost practical importance in severe protracted diarrhoea of infancy. A graduated diagnostic procedure is proposed, taking into account clinical and morphological reactions to cow's milk proteins. Pathogenesis is immunologically mediated. A concept of transient food protein intolerance is developed which has to be separated from the permanent intolerance of gluten in coeliac disease. Prognosis of cow's milk protein intolerance is excellent after elimination of the offending agent. Breast feeding seems to be effective in prevention of the disease.

NEW ENGLAND AND REGIONAL ALLERGY PROCEEDINGS

Heiner DC, Wilson JF "Delayed immunologic food reactions." *N Engl Reg Allergy Proc* (1986 Nov-Dec) 7(6):520-6

Delayed onset reactions to ingested foods may be difficult to recognize, especially if days or weeks elapse before symptoms appear. More than one immunologic mechanism may be involved and it is often difficult to assess the relative importance of each. Because immunologic responses occur in many healthy subjects who readily tolerate a specific food, little importance can be ascribed to a particular immunologic test unless it is shown that at least 95% of normals with similar exposure do not have such a response. Each food contains multiple antigens and allergic individuals differ considerably both in their immune responses and in the clinical manifestations they display. Because of this, the recognition and management of delayed food reactions is complex and requires an awareness of documented food-related disorders. It is a fruitful area for future research.

NAACOGS CLINICAL ISSUES IN PERINATAL AND WOMENS HEALTH NURSING

Walker M "Breastfeeding the premature infant." *NAACOGS Clin Issu Perinat Womens Health Nurs* (1992) 3(4):620-33

Breastfeeding the premature infant is both possible and desirable. Premature infants derive benefits from breast milk that they can not receive from formula. Nutritional issues look at the components of breast milk as they relate to brain growth and development and disease protection in the acute setting and later in childhood. Recommendations for clinical practice are provided, as are information on expressing and collecting milk, breastfeeding readiness, putting the infant to breast, and discharge planning.

Research Appendix

NIPPON JINZO GAKKAI SHI. JAPANESE JOURNAL OF NEPHROLOGY

Yamada T, Nakanishi T, Uyama O, Iida T, Sugita M "[A case of the milk-alkali syndrome with a small amount of milk and magnesium oxide ingestion—the contribution of sustained metabolic alkalosis induced by hypertonic dehydration]" *Nippon Jinzo Gakkai Shi* (1991 Jun) 33(6):581-6 (Published in Japanese)

We described a patient with the milk-alkali syndrome induced by the ingestion of small amount of milk (200 ml/day) and ice cream (145 g/day) and the administration of small dose of absorbable alkali (magnesium oxide 2.0 g/day) for the treatment of chronic constipation. The present case shows not only triads, i.e., hypercalcemia (s-Ca 14.3 mg/dl), metabolic alkalosis (s-HCO3- 37.4 mEq/L), and renal insufficiency (s-Cre 2.3 mg/dl) but also hypernatremia (s-Na 161 mEq/L) and hypertonic dehydration after the frequent episodes of elevated body temperature. The milk-alkali syndrome has been defined as the hypercalcemia with a metabolic alkalosis from a high amount of calcium intake and long term administration of absorbable alkali in any form, usually as calcium carbonate for the treatment of peptic ulcer. As the present case could be distinguished from any other cases previously reported with regard to the amount of calcium (0.4 g/day) and alkali (36 mEq/day) intake and the clinical situations that induced the syndrome, we compared the present case with the previous reports, calculating the amount of calcium and alkali intake from milk and absorbable alkali. After the introduction of the H2 blockers for peptic ulceration, the most cases with milk-alkali syndrome had provoked by the smaller amount of calcium than previously reported, which were associated with the treatment of relatively large amount of alkali (50-150 mEq/day), suggesting the role of sustained metabolic alkalosis for the development. In the present case the metabolic alkalosis induced by hypertonic dehydration and enhanced by absorbable alkali intake also could cause an increase of renal tubular reabsorption of calcium and a decrease of ionized calcium which might produce increased secretion of parathyroid hormone followed by vitamin D3 activation and increased Ca absorption from the gut. The metabolic alkalosis might be essential to the development of the milk-alkali syndrome without a high calcium and absorbable alkali intake.

Institutional address: Fifth Dept. of Internal Medicine
Hyogo College of Medicine.

NUTRICION HOSPITALARIA

Ortega RM, Requejo AM, Andres P, Gaspar MJ, Ortega A "[Milk and dairy products in the prevention and control of cardiovascular diseases] La leche y productos lacteos en la prevencion y control de las enfermedades cardiovasculares." *Nutr Hosp* (1993 Sep-Oct) 8(7):395-404 (Published in Spanish)

Highly saturated fat and cholesterol intakes elevate serum cholesterol levels, which is a risk factor for suffering from cardiovascular disease, one of the most important death causes in developed countries. Milk and dairy products, because of their high saturated fat and cholesterol levels, are often included among the forbidden foodstuffs for people with high serum cholesterol levels. But our studies demonstrate that dairy products, including the whole cream ones, don't increase total cholesterol but increase HDL-cholesterol levels. The intake of skimmed dairy products seem to have a preventive effect on the developing of atherosclerosis, because they condition decreases in serum cholesterol levels, specially in people with hyperlipemia. Dairy products are also effective for the control of triglyceridemia, hypertension and other cardiovascular risk factors. When the dietitian introduces nutritional measurements to prevent or stop cardiovascular disease, it is important to know the nutritional status of the person, in order that the fight against cardiovascular disease does not lead to nutritional deficiencies with similar or worse sanitary repercussions than cardiovascular disease itself. Dairy products are excellent sources of proteins, vitamins and minerals. Their regular intake can prevent, whereas their restriction can lead to nutritional deficit and pathologies. The results of our study show that it is not advisable to limit the intake of dairy products, not even whole cream ones. Only if there is a pathology, as hypercholesterolemia, it can be beneficial to consume skimmed and semi-skimmed dairy products.

Institutional address: Departamento de Nutricion
Facultad de Farmacia Universidad
Complutense Madrid Espa~na.

SCANDINAVIAN JOURNAL OF GASTROENTEROLOGY. SUPPLEMENT

Tamm A "Management of lactose intolerance." *Scand J Gastroenterol Suppl* (1994) 202:55-63

The management of lactose intolerance comprises two parts: (1) the basic principles of treatment in persons intolerant to a dietary dose of lactose, and (2) main manoeuvres to reduce the lactose content in food, and/or consumption of special products of milk or exogenous lactase enzyme. The tactics of management depend on the type of hypolactasia, the severity of intolerance, and on the age of the patient. Special attention is paid to the development of lactose intolerance in some patients via iatrogenic mechanisms such as certain drugs, gastric surgery and ionizing radiation.

Institutional address: Tartu University Estonia.

Villako K, Maaroos H "Clinical picture of hypolactasia and lactose intolerance." *Scand J Gastroenterol Suppl* (1994) 202:36-54

Selective adult-type hypolactasia, the main cause of primary malabsorption of lactose, shows considerable variation in terms of its symptoms, which mainly depend on the amount of milk consumption. The article discusses congenital lactase deficiency and familial lactose intolerance. Links between hypolactasia and non-specific abdominal complaints, coronary heart disease and cataract are presented. The decrease in lactase activity in the brush border of jejunal mucosa, associated with diseases of the mucosa or any other condition which damages the enterocytes, is discussed as a cause of secondary hypolactasia. It is shown that adult-type primary hypolactasia and selective lactose malabsorption represent a major problem in the everyday work of general practitioners, particularly in populations where hypolactasia is common. Therefore, the examination and treatment of non-selected patients with vague abdominal complaints is important in primary health care. As the need for calcium in humans is largely met by the intake of milk, the consumption of milk has to be in amounts that are tolerable for the individual.

Institutional address: University of Tartu Estonia.

REFERENCES AND SUGGESTED READINGS

CHAPTER ONE

Committee on Nutrition, American Academy of Pediatrics: Should milk drinking by children be discouraged? *Pediatrics*, 53:576, 1974

Floch, M.H.: Whither bovine milk? *Amer. J. Clin., Nutr.*, 22:214, 1969

The weaning of America. *Eastwest Journal,* June, 1980, p. 27

There's a fly in the milk bottle. *Medical World News*, May 17, 1974, p. 30.

CHAPTER TWO

Bart RG, Levine MD and Watkins JB: Recurrent abdominal pain of childhood due to lactose intolerance. *N Engl J Med* 300:1449, 1979

Bayless TM and Huang S: Recurrent abdominal pain due to milk and lactose intolerance in school aged children. *Pediatrics* 47:1029, 1971

Bayles TM et al: Lactose and milk intolerance: clinical implications. *N Engl J Med* 292:1156, 1975.

Graham GG: Protein Advisory Group's recommendation deplored. *Pediatrics* 55:295, 1975

Liebman WM: Recurrent abdominal pain in children: lactose and sucrose intolerance, a prospective study. *Pediatrics* 64:43, 1979.

Paige DM et al: Lactose malabsorption and milk rejection in Negro children. *John Hopkins Med J* 129:163, 1971

Simoons FJ, Johnson JD and Kretchmer N: Perspective on milk-drinking and malabsorption of lactose. *Pediatrics* 59:98, 1977.

CHAPTER THREE

Baggett D., Jr: Personal communication.

Bahna SL and Heiner DC: Allergies to milk. New York, Grune and Stratton, 1980.

Deling B et al: Hypersensitivity to foods in steroid-dependent nephrosis. *Clin Res* 74A, 1975

Gerrard JW, Mackenzie JWA, Goluboff N et al: Cow's milk allergy: prevalence and manifestations in an unselected series of newborns. *Acta Paediatr Scand, Supplement 234,* 1973.

Gryboski JD: Gastrointestinal milk allergy in infants. *Pediatrics* 40:354, 1967.

CHAPTER FOUR

Brody JE: Eating less may be the key to living beyond 100 years. *New York Times*, CI, Tuesday, June 8, 1982.

Blumenthal S et al: Risk factors for coronary artery disease in children of affected families. *J Pediatr* 87:1187, 1975.

Diet Nutrition and Cancer. National Academy Press, 1982.

Gilmore CP: "The real villain in heart disease. *New York Times Magazine*, March 25, 1973, p. 31.

Miettinen M et al: Effect of cholesterol lowering diet on mortality from coronary heart disease and other causes. *Lancet* 2:835, 1972.

Osborn GR: Atherosclerosis and infant feeding practices. *Coli Int Centre Nat Scient* 169:93, 1968.

Tsang RC and Glueck CJ: Atherosclerosis: a pediatric perspective. *Curr Prob in Pediatr* 9: No 3, 1979.

CHAPTER FIVE

Barness L: Developmental nutrition: fat. Children are different. No. 5, Ross Laboratories.

Committee on Nutrition, American Academy of Pediatrics: Breast feeding. *Pediatrics* 62:591, 1978.

Cunningham AS: Morbidity in breast-fed and artificially-fed infants. *J Pediatr* 90:726, 1977.

Fomon SJ: Infant Nutrition. Philadelphia, WB Saunders Company. 1975.

Gerard JW: Breast-feeding—second thoughts. *Pediatrics* 54:757, 1974.

Jelliffe DB and Jelliffe EFP: Human milk, nutrition, and the world resource crisis. *Science* 188:557, 1975.

Lepage P, Munyazaki C and Hennart P: Breastfeeding and hospital mortality in children in Ruanda. *Lancet* 2:409, 1981.

Margulies L: Baby formula abroad: exporting infant malnutrition. *Christianity and Crisis,* November 10, 1975, p. 264.

Martinez GA and Dodd DA: 1981 Milk feeding patterns in the United States during the first twelve months of life. *Pediatrics,* 1982 (in press).

Ross CA and Dawes EA: Resistance of the breast-fed infant to gastroenteritis. *Lancet* 1:994, 1954.

CHAPTER SIX

Walker ARP: The human requirement of calcium: should low intakes be supplemented? *Amer J Clin Nutr* 25:518, 1972.

CHAPTER SEVEN

Milk: could it taste better? could it cost less? *Consumer Reports,* June, 1982.

Milk: why is the quality so low? *Consumer Reports,* January, 1974, p. 70.

CHAPTER EIGHT

Agranoff BW and Goldberg D: Diet and the geographical distribution of multiple sclerosis. *Lancet* 2:1061, 1974.

Ferrer JF, Kenyon SJ and Gupta P: Milk of dairy cows frequently contains a leukomogenic virus. *Science* 213:1014, 1981.

Schauss AG and Simonson CE: A critical analysis of the diets of chronic juvenile offenders *J Ortho Psych* 8:149, 179.

CHAPTER NINE

Mackenzie E: Psychologic factors in milk anemia, *Amer Family Physician* 7:80, 1973.

CHAPTER TEN

Crook WG: Food allergy. The great masquerader. *Pediatr Clin No Amer* 22:277, 1975.

Speer F: The allergic tension-fatigue syndrome. *Pediatr Clin No Amer* 1:1029,m 1954.

CHAPTER ELEVEN

Utilization of milk components by the food industry. *Dairy Council Digest* 48:No 5, 1977.

Index

We'd love to send you a free catalog of titles we publish or even to hear your thoughts, reactions, criticisms, about things you did or did not like about this or any other book we publish.

Just write or call us at:

TEACH Services, Inc.
800/367-1998

www.tsibooks.com

ABOUT THE AUTHOR

Frank Oski, born in 1932, is a graduate of Swarthmore College and received his M.D. from the University of Pennsylvania in 1958. He served his internship and Pediatric residency at the Hospital of the University of Pennsylvania and then studied hematology as a Fellow at Harvard at the Boston Children's Hospital. He was appointed as an Associate in the Department of Pediatrics, University of Pennsylvania School of Medicine in 1963 and assumed the post of Professor and Chairman, Department of Pediatrics, State University of New York, Upstate Medical Center in 1972. In 1985 he assumed the position of Director, Department of Pediatrics, Johns Hopkins University School of Medicine and Physician-in-Chief, the Johns Hopkins Children's Center.

Dr. Oski is the author of approximately 290 manuscripts and the author, co-author, editor, or co-editor of 19 textbooks including *Hematologic Problems of the Newborn, Hematology of Infancy and Childhood, The Whole Pediatrician Catalog,* and *Principles and Practice of Pediatrics.*

Dr. Oski has served on the Editorial Board of *Pediatric Research, Pediatrics in Review,* and *Advances in Pediatrics* and was the co-editor of *The Year Book of Pediatrics* from 1976-1991. He serves as the founding and current editor of *Contemporary Pediatrics.*

Dr. Oski has served as a member of the Council of the Society for Pediatric Research and the American Pediatric Society and is the past-president of the Society for Pediatric Research and the president-elect (1991-92) of the American Association of Pediatric Department Chairmen. Dr. Oski is a member of the Society for Pediatric Research, the American Society for Clinical Investigation, the American Pediatric Society, the Association of American Physicians, and the Institute of Medicine, National Academy of Sciences.

Dr. Oski is the recipient of the Mead-Johnson Award for Outstanding Pediatric Research (1972), the St. Geme Award for Pediatric Leadership (1990), the Ross Teaching Award, American Academy of Pediatrics (1990), the Distinguished Graduate Award of the University of Pennsylvania School of Medicine (1990), the Maryland Pediatrician of the Year (1990), and a Doctor of Science (Hon.) from the State University of New York (1991).